From Therapeutic Relationships to Transitional Care

This text provides a foundational understanding of therapeutic relationships and the transitional discharge model (TDM), a person-centered, evidence-based model that supports a smooth transition from hospital to community for people with mental illness.

Starting with background into the ground-breaking work of Dr. Hildegard Peplau, the mother of modern psychiatric nursing, and moving towards a transdisciplinary transitional discharge perspective, chapters introduce students and practitioners to theoretical, historical, and current perspectives on therapeutic relationships as they relate to transitional care. These perspectives foreground empirical research and practical applications that can be implemented in hospital and community settings. The Appendix features an essential "TDM Toolkit" with forms, learning topics, and checklists developed by programs that implement TDM.

Essential reading for those studying psychiatric nursing, this book combines theory, research, and best practices into a "roadmap" for students across nursing and psychiatric disciplines to coordinate these systems without having to implement radical changes to practice.

Cheryl Forchuk, RN, PhD, O Ont, FCAHS, is the Beryl and Richard Ivey Research Chair in Aging, Mental Health, Rehabilitation and Recovery at Parkwood Research Institute and Distinguished Professor at Western University in London, Canada.

From Therapeutic Relationships to Transitional Care

A Theoretical and Practical Roadmap

Edited by

Cheryl Forchuk

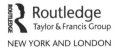

Routledge
Taylor & Francis Group

NEW YORK AND LONDON

First published 2021
by Routledge
52 Vanderbilt Avenue, New York, NY 10017

and by Routledge
2 Park Square, Milton Park, Abingdon, Oxon, OX14 4RN

Routledge is an imprint of the Taylor & Francis Group, an informa business

Library of Congress Cataloging-in-Publication Data
Names: Forchuk, Cheryl, editor.
Title: From therapeutic relationships to transitional care : A theoretical and practical roadmap / edited by Cheryl Forchuk.
Description: New York, NY : Routledge, 2021. | Includes bibliographical references and index. |
Identifiers: LCCN 2020039081 (print) | LCCN 2020039082 (ebook) | ISBN 9780367430399 (paperback) | ISBN 9780367430405 (hardback) | ISBN 9780367430399 (ebook)
Subjects: LCSH: Mental health services. | Nursing care plans.
Classification: LCC RA790 .F76 2021 (print) | LCC RA790 (ebook) | DDC 362.16--dc23
LC record available at https://lccn.loc.gov/2020039081
LC ebook record available at https://lccn.loc.gov/2020039082

ISBN: 978-0-367-43040-5 (hbk)
ISBN: 978-0-367-43039-9 (pbk)
ISBN: 978-1-003-00085-3 (ebk)

Typeset in Times New Roman
by Deanta Global Publishing Services, Chennai, India

About the Cover

The Bridge represents the way forward for a person being discharged from the psychiatric unit (signified by the stark grey building on the left-hand side) to the hopes of a better life in the community (signified by the homes on the green hills on the right-hand side). There is personal support (peer support and/or overlapping staff members) on the bridge reaching out a helping hand, but there are also pillars supporting the bridge that represent family members, friends, healthcare workers, and other staff. Throughout the process of the transitional discharge model studies, whenever participants were asked to visually express their experience, the image of a bridge was a recurring theme. This representation was created to capture the essence of that determination and hope.

Cover art (*The Bridge*) designed by Norma Jean Kelly. The cover art for the book only appears on the paperback edition.

Contents

Conclusion 110

CHERYL FORCHUK

Contributors

Cheryl Forchuk, RN, PhD, O Ont, FCAHS, is the Beryl and Richard Ivey Research Chair in Aging, Mental Health, Rehabilitation and Recovery at Parkwood Research Institute in London, Canada. She is a Distinguished University Professor in nursing and psychiatry at Western University. She is also Assistant Director for the Lawson Health Research Institute, the research arm of both London Health Sciences Centre and St. Joseph's Health Care – London.

Wendy Azzopardi earned her BScN from McMaster University (1988) and MScN from the University of Toronto (1994). She was employed as a staff nurse at Hamilton Psychiatric Hospital (1988–2001) and as a Professor of Nursing in the Conestoga College/McMaster University BScN program (2002–2019). She completed a Spark Fellowship with the Mental Health Commission of Canada (2012–2013) as well as a project at Conestoga College (2017–2019) focusing on Campus Mental Wellness.

Yee-Ching (Lilian) Chan, BBA, CPA, FCMA, PhD, specializes in cost and management accounting. Her research focuses on hospital costing and the application of new management tools in hospitals. She has also conducted research on the performance measurement system and implementation of balanced scorecard in municipal governments. She teaches courses in managerial accounting and controllership at McMaster University in the DeGroote School of Business in Hamilton, Canada.

Raymond Cheng, who with great sadness passed away in January 2019, was involved in testing the transitional discharge model. He served as the Policy Analyst and Knowledge Exchange Facilitator for the Ontario Peer Development Initiative and previously was the Executive Director of a member Consumer/Survivor Initiative in Toronto, Canada. In addition to those roles, he was a board member for the Centre for Addiction and Mental Health and sat on a number of their strategic planning committees. His passion for giving back to the mental health community is commendable.

Deborah Corring has worked in the mental healthcare field since 1972 as a clinician, administrator, researcher, and consultant. She is the owner of a private consultancy firm, Client Perspectives, and is an Adjunct Assistant Professor at Western University for the Department of Psychiatry. Dr. Corring's research interests include projects focused on the use of the transitional discharge model, community treatment orders, and smart technology to support persons with mental illness in the community.

Sebastian Gyamfi, RMN, MPhil, FGCNM, PhD(c), Faculty of Health Sciences, Western University, London, Canada. He has expertise in health promotion and advanced practice in mental health and stigma. He also works at Parkwood Institute of Research with the Mental Health Nursing Research Alliance (MHNRA) in London, Ontario as a Graduate Research Assistant. Sebastian does research in stigma and mental illness, homelessness, structural violence, therapeutic relationships, and community integration.

Boniface Harerimana has PhD and MSc degrees with specialization in addictions science obtained from Western University, Canada and the Institute of Psychiatry, Psychology and Neuroscience at King's College London in the UK, respectively. He has worked for over ten years as both a clinician and program leader in low-resourced and developed countries. He developed and tested the integrated addiction recovery model that advanced healthcare practice and promoted treatment outcomes among individuals with addictions issues.

Margaret Hux, MSc, Dip SP, Health Economist and Registered Psychotherapist (Qualifying) has worked for 20 years for several contract research organizations specializing in health economic and related research for new health technologies becoming integrated into medical practice. As well as research involvements, Margaret is currently establishing a practice in Spiritual Psychotherapy using a range of traditional, somatic, and spiritual modalities for clients with stress, anxiety, depression, and trauma.

Elsabeth Jensen, RN, BA, PhD, is Associate Professor, School of Nursing, at York University in Toronto, Canada. She has authored numerous publications, including book chapters, peer-reviewed papers, and technical reports. Her areas of research expertise are in mental health, childhood abuse, trauma screening, discharge models, program evaluation, and knowledge translation. She is President of the Clinical Nurse Specialist (CNS) Association of Ontario, and President-Elect of the Clinical Nurse Specialist Association of Canada.

Kamini Kalia, RN, MScN, CPMHN(C) is currently the manager for Interprofessional Practice and Education at the Centre for Addiction and Mental Health in Toronto, Canada. In addition to her current role, Kamini has been in various advanced practice nursing leadership and management roles in acute and chronic mental health services in Toronto, London, and St. Thomas. She holds an Adjunct Assistant Professor position in the Arthur Labatt Family School of Nursing at Western University, as well as an Adjunct Clinical Appointment in the Bloomberg Faculty of Nursing at the University of Toronto.

Norma Jean Kelly was the peer support coordinator and advisory group member in projects implementing and testing the transitional discharge model (TDM) as part of her responsibilities at Can Voice, a Consumer/Survivor Initiative. During the following period while providing front-line community mental health services, she also assisted in several arts-based projects involving TDM. She became a registered art therapist in 1997. Although now retired, artmaking continues to be an important part of her life.

Donna Kosterewa-Tolman is a registered nurse who graduated from Mohawk College. Her clinical experience includes general medicine staff nurse, coronary care staff nurse, inpatient psychiatry, and combined inpatient/outpatient geriatric psychiatry and medicine.

Kathleen Ledoux is a nurse who, over the course of her career has been a clinical nurse, a nurse leader, and a nurse academic. Among many accomplishments, Kathleen is most proud of attaining her PhD at a time when she might have contemplated retirement. During her PhD, Kathleen researched the concept of compassion. She has completed the Cultivating Compassion program at Stanford University. Kathleen is an Adjunct Research Professor at Western University.

Amy Lewis is a registered nurse with a Master of Science in Nursing degree from Western University, Canada, and a Graduate Research Assistant of Dr. Cheryl Forchuk at the Lawson Health Research Institute in the Mental Health Nursing Research Alliance.

Brad A. MacNeil, PhD, R. Psych, is a clinical psychologist, consultant, and researcher. He is the Provincial Clinical Leader – Manager Educational & Training Competencies, Policy and Planning with the Nova Scotia Health Authority Mental Health and Addictions Program. He is also an Assistant Professor (Adjunct) in the Department of Psychiatry at Dalhousie University where he provides supervision in cognitive behavior therapy.

Mary-Lou Martin is a clinical nurse specialist in mental health in the Forensic Program at St. Joseph's Healthcare in Hamilton, Canada. She also holds an appointment as an Associate Clinical Professor at McMaster University, School of Nursing. She is President of the Clinical Nurse Specialist Association of Canada.

William Reynolds, PhD, has had a long professional career as a clinician, teacher, researcher, and theorist in several countries and four continents. The main focus of his research was the development and measurement of empathy. His contribution to research and the theories that underpin the therapeutic relationship has been widely disseminated in academic journals, seminars, and keynote speeches. He is appreciative of the mentorship received from Dr. Hildegard Peplau, who taught him how to think.

Abraham (Rami) Rudnick, MD, PhD, MCIL, is a psychiatrist and a philosopher. He is a Professor in the Department of Psychiatry and the School of Occupational Therapy at Dalhousie University and the Clinical Director of the Nova Scotia Operational Stress Injury Clinic, Canada. He is also a member of the Rotman Institute of Philosophy at Western University in Ontario, Canada. He is a recipient of national (Canadian) and international awards and other recognitions for his clinical academic mental health work.

Deborrah Sherman was involved in TDM research projects as Executive Director of Mental Health Rights Coalition of Hamilton first, then Ontario Peer Development Initiative (OPDI). Previously, Deborrah sat on the Consent and Capacity Board in Ontario and taught a Psychosocial Rehabilitation course with Mohawk College. She remains involved with OPDI as a Peer Support Core Essentials trainer. Deborrah also remains an active Certified Peer Supporter and Certified Mentor with Peer Support Canada.

Michelle Solomon is a registered nurse with experience in outpatient and acute mental health care. She is a PhD student in Nursing at Western University with a focus on the role of psychosocial supports in the management of mood disorders. Michelle enjoys program development, is a previous founder of a consumer/survivor organization and director for ten years, and a past facilitator of a youth wellness hub for mental health and addictions.

Rani Srivastava is the Dean, School of Nursing at Thompson Rivers University, Kamloops BC. Formerly, she was Chief of Nursing and Professional Practice at the Centre for Addiction and Mental Health (CAMH) in Toronto. She is passionate about quality patient- and family-centered care for culturally diverse and marginalized populations and is recognized for her leadership and scholarship in diversity, equity, cultural competence, cultural identity, religion, ethics, and family-centered care.

Shirley Tran is a registered nurse at Canadian Mental Health Association, Middlesex, and St. Joseph's Health Care, London. Additionally, she is a Master of Science in Nursing student at Western University, Canada, and a Graduate Research Assistant at the Lawson Health

Research Institute in the Mental Health Nursing Research Alliance, receiving mentorship from Dr. Cheryl Forchuk.

Tazim Virani, RN, BScN, MScN, PhD, is a Registered Nurse in Ontario, Canada, with over 35 years of clinical, system leadership, education, and research experiences. Her research work focused on uptake and sustainability of best practice guidelines at the organization and system levels. Tazim has dedicated her career to improving the nursing profession and patient care by establishing national and international programs in evidence-based practices, participating in system level transformation in mental health, community-based care, and global health.

Jan Westwell obtained her BScN from Laurentian University in 1978 and her MScN from the University of Toronto in 1983. She worked as a clinical nurse specialist at Hamilton Psychiatric Hospital and was an Assistant Professor at McMaster University. Following a career in nursing, she went into business with her husband.

Acknowledgements

Many people assisted in the development of the ideas presented in this book.

I would like to first acknowledge my mentor in understanding therapeutic relationships, Dr. Hildegard Peplau. The correspondence and discussions over the years helped shape my thinking and her work is foundational to this book.

The development of the transitional discharge model would not have been possible without my former colleagues at what was then the Hamilton Psychiatric Hospital. In my work on therapeutic relationships I learned that people generally know what the problems are, and what the solutions might be, but often feel blocked from implementing the solutions. The hospital administration backed my vision that the same could be true on a larger system level – the patients in the hospital and the front-line staff knew the issues and solutions but did not feel empowered to act. The staff and patients on D2, the pilot ward, took a risk in believing we could do things a new way. It would not have been possible to develop and later, more broadly, test this new approach to transitional care without their help.

Similarly, the Mental Health Rights Coalition of Hamilton, a consumer/survivor initiative, took the first steps with us in developing the peer support component. This work was later supported by the Ontario Peer Development Initiative of Ontario, which is an umbrella organization for peer groups across our province. Multiple consumer organizations in Canada and abroad have helped in the implementation of the transitional discharge model.

My research program would not have been possible without the support of fantastic research staff that I have consistently had over the years, including research coordinators, research assistants, and graduate students. With this book, I had a lot of pragmatic assistance from graduate research assistants Amy Lewis, Shirley Tran, and Ivy Tran.

Finally, I would like to thank my children, Ian Forchuk Smits, Robin Forchuk Smits, and Callista Smits Forchuk, who remind me regularly of the importance of family relationships as therapeutic relationships. My children all had times when they accompanied me to various countries and provinces in relation to my work. I will always remember what my youngest (Callie) said when she was around ten and it was near the end of a three-week trip to several countries in Europe. She had gone to school with a daughter of a colleague in Finland and attended gymnastics and a Halloween-type party in Scotland with the daughter of another colleague (so I hadn't made her only attend lectures). However, as preparing to head home she said – "Don't worry Mom – if you ever get laryngitis, I think I have heard this stuff enough I could just give the lecture."

Cheryl Forchuk

About the Book

Within this book, you will find a collection of essays that takes the reader from some of the theoretical origins of therapeutic relationships in the delivery of mental healthcare to practical applications in the transitional discharge model.

Therapeutic relationships are the foundation for all healthcare. This book highlights theory, research, and best practices. The theoretical perspectives are rooted in the ground-breaking work of Dr. Hildegard Peplau, the mother of modern psychiatric nursing. She championed the idea of the client as a partner in the recovery process by speaking of doing "with" rather than doing "to"; in the 1950s, this approach was revolutionary. My early work tested this theory and looked at its application to mental healthcare. The first part of the book covers material on varying aspects of the therapeutic relationship and its major concepts.

The transition from hospital to the community is a critical time for mental stability and potential rehospitalization. To address the many challenges that people face after they are discharged from psychiatric inpatient units, the transitional discharge model (TDM) seeks to preserve relationships with hospital staff until new ones have been fostered with staff from community care organizations. This model is grounded in a relational approach to support the transition between care providers and care agencies. To further help clients during this critical period, the TDM uses a network of peer supporters who have already successfully transitioned into the community. This model of care is theoretically grounded and has reliably produced positive health outcomes for clients, as well as for healthcare systems (Forchuk, Martin, Chan, & Jensen, 2005; Forchuk et al., 2012; Reynolds et al., 2004). A considerable amount of research has been conducted on the effects of discharge on psychiatric clients, but evidence-based models that coordinate health and community systems for successful discharge are limited in number. The utility of the TDM is that it does not require organizations to implement radical change – it is designed to coordinate existing systems with foundational practices that can be applied to a variety of settings. The transitional discharge work moves from seeing the work of Dr. Peplau and others from a nursing perspective to a transdisciplinary perspective.

This book covers the issues of therapeutic relationships and transitional discharge in five parts, each dedicated to a theme: Theoretical Perspectives, Care Recipient Perspectives, Care Provider Perspectives, Exploration of Key Concepts, and From Therapeutic Relationships to Transitional Care.

Cheryl Forchuk
Brantford, Ontario

Part I

Theoretical Perspectives

The theoretical perspectives are rooted in the ground-breaking research of Dr. Hildegard Peplau, the mother of modern psychiatric nursing. I was introduced to Dr. Peplau's work as an undergraduate, but it was not until I completed my master's degree and began my work as a clinical nurse specialist (CNS) that I truly began to understand its significance. I was the sole CNS for a large tertiary care facility that had ten inpatient programs and ten community programs when I started in 1980 at Hamilton Psychiatric Hospital, Ontario, Canada. Given this breadth, I primarily worked on a consultation basis with complex situations where the usual care provided by expert nurses and other staff was simply not working. I was brought in as a fresh set of eyes and ears to meet with the client, care team, and, usually, family to make suggestions and follow up as needed. I would generally have at least two new consultations a week, with follow-up lasting for a month to a year, depending on the situation.

After the first year, I did an analysis of the first 100 consultations and found that close to 80% of consultations were related to the therapeutic relationship (interestingly, about 10% of issues were related to a diversity of sexuality issues, including abuse and identity; the remaining 10% were complex clinical issues, such as an unusual combination of comorbidities or a rare condition). I felt perplexed by the large number of concerns relating to such a basic nursing concept as the therapeutic relationship, especially among highly skilled nurses. This inquiry drew me back to Dr. Peplau's work.

I re-read the original work by Dr. Peplau and reviewed the series of 20 audiotapes she had produced, as well as a videotaped simulated interview she created. These resources were very helpful in assisting with the issues I was encountering in practice. In early 1983, we invited Dr. Peplau to our hospital for three days. Although she was well into her 70s by that point, she was fully booked until April 1984.

We had a full agenda for Dr. Peplau's visit, with lots of time for dialogue. At the end of the visit she said that she was very impressed with the caliber of nursing care, said, "write me," and then gave me her home address. I was eight months pregnant with my second child and shortly after the visit took maternity leave. I honestly was a bit intimidated by the idea of simply writing to the mother of modern psychiatric nursing, so I didn't write. At Christmas (I was still on maternity leave), I received a call from the hospital that I had a Christmas card from Dr. Peplau and was asked if someone lived nearby to drop it off. The card essentially said, "Merry Christmas – you didn't write," and urged me to write back. So, I wrote back and maintained a regular correspondence that lasted until her death in 1990 (I have two very fat binders of all her letters). We were able to meet a few times over those years, as well as have phone calls, and she connected me with many other nursing scholars.

One of the first things she did in her letters was suggest I needed to get a PhD in nursing. I thought I had an iron-clad excuse: I had two children under the age of three, and there was no PhD program in nursing in Canada at that time. She basically said – "Stop making excuses. Kids are easier to manage when younger and you will never get PhD programs in nursing in Canada until enough of you get one outside of the country." So, after some well-intended badgering, I eventually started my PhD at Wayne State in Detroit in 1987, graduating in 1992.

Chapter 1 in this book gives an overview of Peplau's theory. You will see the references to personal communication in this book that reflect our conversations about having her theory look more like a theory, which needed to include a picture. The diagram illustrating her theory in that chapter went back and forth many times between us until she was happy that it was an accurate picture. I was very happy when she later told me that she had it translated into Japanese for presentations in Japan about her theory! Some of this material originally was in a small booklet published by Sage as a series on nursing theorists in 1993 [Forchuk, C. (1993). *Hildegard E. Peplau: Interpersonal nursing theory*. SAGE Publications]. The copyright reverted to me after it went out of print. It has been revised and updated as a chapter in this book.

Chapter 2 in this book is a republication of a paper of the main findings from my PhD thesis, which tested Peplau's theory [Forchuk, C. (1994). The orientation phase of the nurse-client relationship: Testing Peplau's theory. *Journal of Advanced Nursing, 20*(3), 532–537. https://doi.org/10.1111/j.1365-2648.1994.tb02392.x]. This work flowed from the hypotheses of the theory as described in the first chapter. The idea that both the nurse and client are important partners in the relationship was validated. Central concepts in the theory can predict the development of the therapeutic relationship.

1   Overview of Peplau's Theory

Cheryl Forchuk

Hildegard Peplau is a nursing pioneer and the mother of modern psychiatric-mental health nursing practice (see Table 1.1). Peplau stated that she began her theory development in response to

> the need in the late 1940s to develop "advanced psychiatric nursing" for graduate programs in psychiatric nursing. The available nursing literature in psychiatric nursing at that time was not in any way adequate for graduate level, university-based psychiatric nursing education programs.
>
> (personal correspondence, December 23, 1990)

Her original intent was not theory development, but "only to convey to the nursing profession ideas [she] thought were important to improve practice" (personal correspondence, July 1989).

Peplau's (1952) first book, *Interpersonal Relations in Nursing*, was published in 1952 and reissued in 1988 and 1991. This book outlined her conceptual framework for psychodynamic nursing. Peplau's conceptual framework signified the end of a long drought in the development of nursing theory as it was the first published nursing theory development since Nightingale.

Origins of the Theory

Dr. Peplau first studied interpersonal relations theory in the 1930-1940s at Bennington College (personal correspondence, December 23, 1990). This interpersonal focus underpinned her later theory development.

Peplau was strongly influenced by the interpersonal development model of Harry Stack Sullivan (1952) and incorporated his theory of personality development and the self-system in her work. Peplau, like Sullivan, was also influenced by the early work of symbolic interactionists such as George Hubert Mead (1934). Examples of the influence of symbolic interactionism can be seen in the focus on social influences on personal development and with the idea that communication involves the use of symbols. Other influences include Rallo May's (1950) work on anxiety and the understanding of learning developed by Miller and Dollard (1941).

Peplau's 1952 work was grounded in interpersonal theory and the clinical experiences of herself and students. Peplau stated "… concepts emerged from practice – my own and supervisory review of graduate student nurses beginning in 1948 – from actual nurse-patient relationship data" (personal correspondence, August 1989).

Table 1.1 Biographical Sketch of a Nurse Theorist: Hildegard E. Peplau

Born	September 1, 1909
Position	Professor Emerita, Rutgers University
Registered Nurse	Pottstown, Pennsylvania Hospital School of Nursing
B.A.	Interpersonal psychology, Bennington College, Vermont
M.A.	Teaching and supervision of psychiatric nursing Teacher's College, Columbia University
Ed.D.	Teacher's College, Columbia University, New York, New York
Fellow	American Academy of Nursing
Other	Honorary Doctorates from University of Indianapolis, Rutgers University, Columbia University, Duke University, Boston College and Alfred University; and numerous other honors.
Died	March 17, 1999 in Sherman Oaks, California. She was in her 90th year.

Forchuk, C. (1993). *Hildegard E. Peplau: Interpersonal nursing theory.* SAGE Publications.

Since 1952, Peplau was a prolific writer. She published a second book in 1964, dictated a series of 20 audiotapes to teach and communicate her theory, and published more than 80 chapters and articles. Her work has endured over the years and is widely used in clinical practice. Sills (1978) reviewed several prominent nursing journals and found that references to Peplau's work had not only been sustained, but actually increased over the years.

In the late 1980s, two Canadian surveys (Martin & Kirkpatrick, 1987, 1989) found that in a tertiary care psychiatric hospital, approximately two-thirds of the nursing staff used Peplau's theory as a basis for their practice. Similarly, an American survey (Hirschmann, 1989) of mental health nurses in private practice found that approximately half were guided by Peplau's theory. With less emphasis on nursing theory in recent years, more recent surveys were not found; however, chapters in current psychiatric-mental health nursing texts still refer to her body of work as foundational (Austin et al., 2013; Halter, 2014; Wright & McKeown, 2018). Current guidelines, such as the Registered Nurses' Association of Ontario (RNAO, 2002/2006) best practice guideline *Establishing Therapeutic Relationships* and RNAO (2017) *Nurse Educator Mental Health and Addiction Resource* incorporate her work.

Although Peplau's theory has been most frequently used by psychiatric or mental health nurses, Peplau believed that psychodynamic nursing transcended all clinical nursing specialties and that all nursing is based on the interpersonal process and the relationship that develops between the nurse and client.

Assumptions of the Theory

Assumptions are basic beliefs with a given theory that are accepted as true. One must accept the given assumptions of a theory in order to adopt it. The concepts are the major components or building blocks of the theory.

In Peplau's 1952 book, she identified two "guiding assumptions" as underpinnings to her framework. These were:

1. "The kind of nurse each person becomes makes a substantial difference in what each client will learn as she or he is nursed through her or his experience with illness" (p. xi).
2. "Fostering personality development in the direction of maturity is a function of nursing and nursing education; it requires the use of principles and methods that permit and guide the process of grappling with everyday interpersonal problems or difficulties" (p. xi).

Peplau (1989c; personal correspondence, December 1990) also stated as assumptions that:

3. "Nursing can take as its unique focus the reactions of clients to the circumstances of their illness or health problems" (1989c, p. 28).
4. "Since illness provides an opportunity for learning and growth, nursing can assist clients to gain intellectual and interpersonal competencies, beyond those that they have at the point of illness, by gearing nursing practices to evolving such competencies through nurse-client interactions" (1989c, p. 28). Peplau references Gregg (1954) and Mereness (1966) in the development of this fourth assumption.

Additional implicit and explicit assumptions by Forchuk (1991) include:

5. "Psychodynamic nursing crosses all specialty areas of nursing. It is not synonymous with psychiatric nursing since every nurse-client relationship is an interpersonal situation in which recurring difficulties of everyday life arise" (summarized from Peplau, 1952, introduction).
6. "Difficulties in interpersonal relations recur in varying intensities throughout the life of everyone" (Peplau, 1952, p. xiv).
7. "The need to harness energy that derives from tension and anxiety connected to felt needs to positive means for defining, understanding, and meeting productively the problem at hand is a universal need" (Peplau, 1952, p. 26).
8. "All human behavior is purposeful and goal-seeking in terms of feelings of satisfaction and/or security" (Peplau, 1952, p. 86).
9. "The interaction of nurse and client is fruitful when a method of communication that identifies and uses common meanings is at work in the situation" (Peplau, 1952, p. 284)
10. "The meaning of behavior to the client is the only relevant basis on which nurses can determine needs to be met" (Peplau, 1952, p. 226).
11. "Each person will behave, during any crisis, in a way that has worked in relation to crises faced in the past" (Peplau, 1952, p. 255).

Concepts of the Theory

Peplau's theory focuses on the interpersonal processes and therapeutic relationship that develops between the nurse and client. Figure 1.1 depicts the major concepts of Peplau's theory within this interpersonal perspective.

The metaparadigm, or concepts, of nursing includes nursing, person, environment, and health. Peplau's theory defines the concepts of the metaparadigm in the following way:

1. "*Nursing* is an educative instrument, a maturing force, that aims to promote health" (Peplau, 1952).
2. "*Person* is an individual, developed through interpersonal relationships, that lives in an unstable environment" (Peplau, 1952).
3. "*Environment* is physiological, psychological, social fluidity that may be illness-maintaining or health-promoting" (Peplau, 1952, 1973c, 1987).
4. "*Health* is forward movement of personality and other on-going human processes in the direction of creative and constructive personal and community living" (Peplau, 1952).

Interpersonal Focus

The interpersonal focus of Peplau's theory requires that the nurse attend to the interpersonal processes that occur between the nurse and client. This is in sharp contrast to many nursing

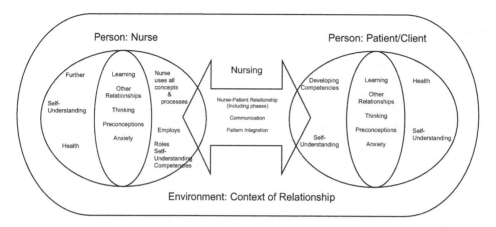

Figure 1.1 Peplau's Framework: Major Concepts and Their Relationships. Forchuk, C. (1993). *Hildegard E. Peplau: Interpersonal nursing theory.* Sage Publications.

theories that focus on the client as the unit of attention. Although individual client factors are assessed, the nurse also self-reflects. The focus is the interpersonal process and relationships, not the constituent parts (or individuals). Interpersonal processes include: the nurse–client relationship, communication, pattern integration, and the roles of the nurse.

Nurse–Client Relationship

Peplau's interpersonal theory of nursing identifies the therapeutic nurse–client relationship as the crux of nursing. The nurse–client relationship evolves through identifiable, overlapping phases. The phases include orientation, working, and resolution. The Relationship Form (see Figure 1.2), developed by Forchuk et al. (1986) and tested by Forchuk and Brown (1989), gives a pictorial overview of the nurse and client behaviors at each phase. The reliability and validity of the form was reported in Forchuk and Brown (1989). An updated version of the form including therapeutic and non-therapeutic relationships is included in the TDM toolkit in this book.

The initial phase of the nurse–client relationship is the orientation phase where the nurse and client come to know each other as persons and the client begins to trust the nurse. The time in the orientation phase can vary from a few minutes of the initial meeting to months of regular sessions.

The second phase of the nurse–client relationship, the working phase, is subdivided into identification and exploitation subphases. In the identification subphase the client begins to identify problems to be worked on within the relationship. The nature of the problems identified can be as diverse as the scope of nursing practice. Examples include identifying inadequate pain management, requests for health teaching regarding breast feeding, or wanting to discuss unresolved issues related to past sexual abuse. The exploitation subphase occurs as the client makes use of the services of the nurse to work through the identified problems. Often, as initial problems are worked through, further problems are identified by the client.

The nurse does not "solve" the client's problems, but rather gives the client the opportunity to explore options and possibilities within the context of the relationship. For example, the

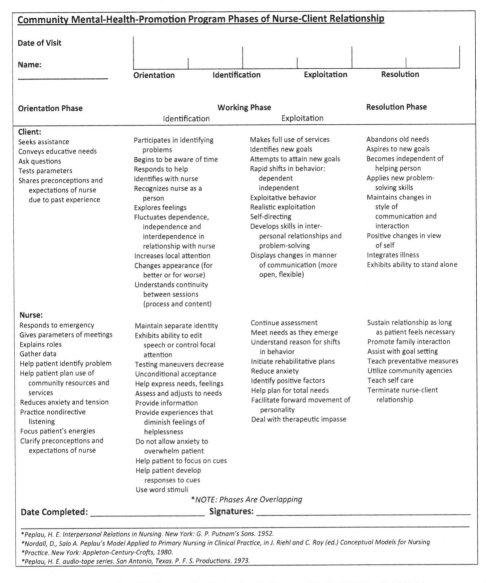

Community Mental-Health-Promotion Program Phases of Nurse-Client Relationship

Orientation Phase	**Working Phase**	**Resolution Phase**
	Identification / Exploitation	
Client:		
Seeks assistance	Participates in identifying problems	Makes full use of services	Abandons old needs

Client:

Orientation Phase	Identification	Exploitation	Resolution Phase
Seeks assistance	Participates in identifying problems	Makes full use of services	Abandons old needs
Conveys educative needs	Begins to be aware of time	Identifies new goals	Aspires to new goals
Ask questions	Responds to help	Attempts to attain new goals	Becomes independent of helping person
Tests parameters	Identifies with nurse	Rapid shifts in behavior: dependent independent	Applies new problem-solving skills
Shares preconceptions and expectations of nurse due to past experience	Recognizes nurse as a person	Exploitative behavior	Maintains changes in style of communication and interaction
	Explores feelings	Realistic exploitation	
	Fluctuates dependence, independence and interdependence in relationship with nurse	Self-directing	Positive changes in view of self
	Increases local attention	Develops skills in interpersonal relationships and problem-solving	Integrates illness
	Changes appearance (for better or for worse)	Displays changes in manner of communication (more open, flexible)	Exhibits ability to stand alone
	Understands continuity between sessions (process and content)		

Nurse:

Orientation Phase	Identification	Exploitation	Resolution Phase
Responds to emergency	Maintain separate identity	Continue assessment	Sustain relationship as long as patient feels necessary
Gives parameters of meetings	Exhibits ability to edit speech or control focal attention	Meet needs as they emerge	Promote family interaction
Explains roles		Understand reason for shifts in behavior	Assist with goal setting
Gather data	Testing maneuvers decrease	Initiate rehabilitative plans	Teach preventative measures
Help patient identify problem	Unconditional acceptance	Reduce anxiety	Utilize community agencies
Help patient plan use of community resources and services	Help express needs, feelings	Identify positive factors	Teach self care
Reduces anxiety and tension	Assess and adjusts to needs	Help plan for total needs	Terminate nurse-client relationship
Practice nondirective listening	Provide information	Facilitate forward movement of personality	
Focus patient's energies	Provide experiences that diminish feelings of helplessness	Deal with therapeutic impasse	
Clarify preconceptions and expectations of nurse	Do not allow anxiety to overwhelm patient		
	Help patient to focus on cues		
	Help patient develop responses to cues		
	Use word stimuli		

NOTE: Phases Are Overlapping

Date of Visit — Orientation / Identification / Exploitation / Resolution

Date Completed: _____ **Signatures:** _____

*Peplau, H. E. Interpersonal Relations in Nursing. New York: G. P. Putnam's Sons. 1952.
*Nordall, D., Salo A. Peplau's Model Applied to Primary Nursing in Clinical Practice, in J. Riehl and C. Roy (ed.) Conceptual Models for Nursing
*Practice. New York: Appleton-Century-Crofts, 1980.
*Peplau, H. E. audio-tape series. San Antonio, Texas. P. F. S. Productions. 1973.

Figure 1.2 The Relationship Form. Forchuk, C., & Brown, B. E. (1989). Establishing a nurse-client relationship. *Psychosocial Nursing, 27*(2), 30–34. https://doi.org/10.3928/0279-3695-19890201-10

nurse may provide information on community resources, or provide health teaching related to medication, illness, or health promotion if appropriate in the context of the relationship; however, the nurse employing Peplau's theory would resist all temptation related to "advice giving" because this would undermine the roles and responsibilities of the client.

The resolution phase of the relationship occurs between the time actual problems are resolved and the time the relationship is terminated. Examples of work that may need to be done in this period include connecting the client to community resources, working through dependency issues in the relationship, learning preventative measures, strengthening social supports, and summarizing the work completed.

The nurse–client relationship does not evolve as a simple linear process. Although the relationship may be predominantly in one phase, reflections of all phases can be seen in each interaction. Every interaction has a beginning (orientation), middle (working), and end (resolution) that reflect the larger pattern of the ongoing nurse–client relationship.

Communication

Communication includes both verbal communication and non-verbal communication. Verbal communication is expressed through language, while non-verbal communication is expressed through empathic linkages, gestures, postures, and patterns.

Verbal communication, or language, is important as a reflection of thought processes. This is obvious on the literal content level: For example, the client gives information on pain, on current abilities, or on perceptions of problems. In addition to the literal content, there are symbolic meanings, patterns, and underlying assumptions that can be conveyed through the choice of words or phrases. Consider the difference among the following statements: "I have a chronic migraine headache problem and it appears to be starting to flare up," "My head is killing me," and "I'm getting a headache." Different information is conveyed regarding ownership of the headache, possible intellectualizing, and degree of distress; however, one would not make immediate assumptions, but rather be attentive to emerging patterns and validate these with the client (or better yet, encourage the client to note the patterns and validate these with the nurse).

Peplau considers the use of verbal communication to be an essential component of the nurse–client relationship. She states, "The general principle is that anything clients act out with nurses will most probably not be talked about, and that which is not discussed cannot be understood" (1989a, p. 197). Talking about issues and concerns gives the client an alternative to acting out these issues.

Peplau (1973d) has described patterns of word usage that may require corrective action on the part of the nurse. Common patterns include:

1. Overgeneralization – For example, the client says, "The worst things always happen to me." The nurse would attempt to help the client be more specific by asking for one incident.
2. Inappropriate use of pronouns – A paranoid client may insist "they" are out to get him, and the nurse asks, "Who are they?"
3. The suggestion of automatic knowing through repetition of the phrase "you know" – The nurse conveys the information that "I only know what you tell me about it," and drops such phrases from his or her language.

This corrective use of language is quite similar to approaches suggested by cognitive therapists such as Aaron Beck (1976) and Albert Ellis (1962). A difference is that cognitive therapy assumes one is directly changing the thought. Peplau believes one is changing the language, but because thought and language are part of an integral whole, a change in one is reflected in the other.

Non-verbal language is more subtle than verbal language and may at times contradict the verbal message. Consider the example of the person who screams, "I am not upset!" In such cases it is the non-verbal message that tends to be believed. Congruence is an important consideration for the nurse to monitor in his or her own communication. Empathy and caring can be transmitted on a non-verbal level as can feelings, such as indifference or hostility.

Most non-verbal communication is culturally influenced, so one must be cautious in transcultural interpretation and use of gestures. For example, does avoiding eye contact suggest dishonesty, shyness, or respect? It can depend on the cultural orientations of the sender and receiver of the message.

A personal example that exemplifies the need for an awareness of cultural differences occurred in the author's work with an Indigenous person. I had concerns about how the sessions were progressing. The client stated he felt things were going well. I could not identify what was bothering me but thought the problem might be culturally related. The client and I had one session video-taped to be viewed by a cultural anthropologist. The client and I viewed the videotape with the anthropologist, and we all noticed the almost comical "dance of the eyes." He was attempting to avoid eye contact as I was attempting to maintain it. We discussed our different interpretations of eye contact (he avoided eye contact in deference to authority and out of respect, while I believed I was trying to maintain our open communication through eye contact). We agreed to not impose our rules on each other; however, the client noted that every time he went for a promotion interview, he was unsuccessful, and that the feedback I had given prior to the tape about "something not seeming quite right" was similar to the feedback he received after the interviews. He decided to use eye contact in job interview/promotion situations. Although I believe his success reflected more than a change in eye contact, that client was convinced that the two promotions he received in the next year were related to his new awareness of this difference in communication. This situation also exemplifies how learning in the nurse–client relationship can be used in other relationships, and that both the nurse and client learn and grow in the therapeutic relationship.

Similar examples of non-verbal communications that can be interpreted very differently by different people include touching, hugging, smiling, passing flatulence, hand movements, comfortable social distances, crossing legs, gestures, offering food, and gift-giving. These acts can have vastly different cultural meanings to different groups and individuals. Therefore, the nurse needs to be aware of issues related to differences in interpretation of non-verbal communication when providing care to a client from a different cultural group. The nurse, through self-reflection and clinical supervision, also needs to be aware of his or her own personal and cultural non-verbal patterns that might, at times, interfere with the evolving nurse–client relationship.

Pattern Integration

Each individual and each system has customary patterns of interacting with others. Pattern integrations are the products of the interaction of the patterns of more than one individual or system. Peplau (1973c, 1987) has identified four common pattern integrations: complementary, mutual, antagonistic, and mixed.

A *complementary* pattern integration involves patterns that are different yet fit together like parts of a jigsaw puzzle. The "fit" assists in ensuring the continuity of the single patterns that make up the integration. An example of this integration can be found with the nurse who insists on "helping" clients by doing things they could actually do for themselves. This could range from cutting their meat at dinner to arranging an out-patient appointment. A complementary pattern occurs when this nurse works with a dependent client who prefers that others make all possible decisions. The nurse and client will form a comfortable partnership that will make it difficult for either to change. A similar integration could be perpetuated on a larger systems level if this dyad worked in the context of a hospital that emphasized the accountability of the nurse but not the accountability or involvement in decision making of the client. Similar examples of complementary pattern integrations include anger-withdrawal, domination-submission, and belittling-others–belittling-self.

A *mutual* pattern integration occurs when two or more interacting individuals/systems display a similar pattern. The multiple use of a single pattern also assists in the continuity of each similar pattern. A classic example from the nursing literature is the mutual-withdrawal pattern first identified by Gwen Tudor (1952/1970) as occurring between specific clients and staff on an inpatient psychiatric unit. Unfortunately, examples of this mutual pattern can still be found across nursing specialties: consider the placement of selected, less desirable, medical or surgical patients as far away from the nursing station as possible, or the early discharge of some community clients who give the impression they are not interested in interacting with the nurse, despite their ongoing personal health problems.

Additional examples of mutual pattern integrations include mutual anger, mutual disrespect, and mutual self-denigration. Positive examples include mutual respect or mutual concern. It is important to consider that the nurse should employ mutual pattern integrations only with those patterns that the nurse and client would want to perpetuate.

Antagonistic pattern integrations include the combination of different individual patterns that do not fit well together. The combination, therefore, creates a discomfort or disharmony that can be used as a motivation toward change. An example given by Peplau (1973c) is that of a client with an angry pattern with a nurse who is using an investigative approach ("Tell me about what's going on") rather than responding with a complementary (e.g., withdrawal) or mutual (e.g., also responding in anger) pattern. Obviously, this is the ideal integration for patterns that require change.

The antagonistic pattern can also occur at an individual or larger systems levels. An example of an antagonistic pattern at the larger systems level could occur with a client who feels most comfortable being dependent and letting others "take care" of him or her. An antagonistic pattern would emerge if this client was in a therapeutic environment that encouraged the participation and decision making of all individuals. It would become uncomfortable for the client to maintain dependent behaviors.

An even broader systems example of an antagonistic pattern would be the introduction of a nursing care delivery system that emphasizes the accountability of each nurse (e.g., primary nursing) into a traditional paternalistic hospital system. The traditional paternalistic system emphasizes centralized decision making rather than decision making and accountability at the staff level. Thus, the nursing care delivery system would create an antagonistic pattern with the larger hospital system. If change is desired, it would be beneficial for the antagonistic pattern integration to occur as frequently as possible and at a variety of personal and larger systems levels.

Other examples of antagonistic pattern integrations include withdrawal-seeking out, dependence-promoting independence, and self-denigration-acceptance of self and others. It needs to be remembered that the inherent incongruence of antagonistic pattern integrations is anxiety producing. The resultant anxiety needs to be harnessed and channeled toward change; however, the anxiety also requires careful monitoring so that it does not become overwhelming. This issue is more fully addressed under the concept of anxiety.

Peplau (1987) has also identified *mixed* or changing pattern integrations. These include a combination of the earlier identified pattern integrations. For example, a person may respond to another's anger by first getting angry themselves (reflecting a mutual pattern integration) and then withdrawing (reflecting a complementary pattern). Mutual-complementary combinations continue to reinforce individual patterns. Antagonistic pattern integration used in combination with a mutual or complementary integration will lose effectiveness in promoting change, since individuals are more likely to respond to patterns that reinforce familiar and comfortable personal patterns.

Roles of the Nurse

The nurse may enact several roles with the client. The roles depend on the needs of the client and the skills and creativity of the nurse. The possible roles will also be influenced by the nurse's position and agency policies. For example, a community nurse in a case management program may include a role related to cutting through red tape in order to ensure that appropriate services are in place for the client. A clinical nurse specialist may include roles that allow the nurse to transcend institutional or agency boundaries. An example includes following a client through different hospital and community settings. On the other hand, a staff nurse working a set shift may find more limitations to the type of roles they can offer to the client. The nurse needs to be aware of the possibilities and constraints so that accurate information can be conveyed to the client.

Peplau's (1952) book includes the following examples of roles: stranger, resource person, teacher, leader, surrogate for significant others, counselor, arbitrator, change-agent, researcher, and technical expert. Regardless of other roles assumed, the nurse and client always begin the relationship as strangers to each other.

In her 1964 book, Peplau emphasized the importance of the counselor role and stated that this was the primary role to be undertaken by nurses in psychiatric-mental health nursing. Traditionally, psychiatric nurses focused on surrogate roles, particularly parent surrogate roles, and the result was custodial care that minimized the potential for growth and change. Peplau (1964) stated, "If [nurses] are unable to contribute in a truly corrective manner to the care of mental patients, the traditional nurse-patient relationship will be usurped by those who can; and the nurses will be shunted into the role of glorified custodian or superclerk" (p. 7).

The counselor role must be valued as the prime vehicle for the development of the nurse–client relationship. Frequently this involves individual counseling. Other modes, such as group work, community development, and family systems nursing, are also appropriate. Within these modalities, the group, community, or family would be the "client" rather than the individual as the client; the nurse–client relationship would develop in phases; and the concepts of communication, both verbal and non-verbal, pattern integrations, and roles of the nurse would also be applicable.

Intrapersonal Processes

Although the primary focus within Peplau's theory is on *inter*personal processes, *intra*personal processes of both the client and nurse are also considered. Intrapersonal processes are processes that occur within the person, rather than between people. There is a strong interrelationship between interpersonal and intrapersonal phenomena: intrapersonal structures, processes, and changes develop through interpersonal activity. Examples of intrapersonal concepts within Peplau's theory include anxiety, learning, thinking, and competencies. Although each of these is observed on an individual level, these concepts have interpersonal implications.

Anxiety

Anxiety is an energy that emerges in response to a perceived threat. The threat can range from the physical to the metaphysical. Peplau (1989a) described the sequence of steps in the development of anxiety as including "holding expectations, expectations not met, discomfort felt, relief behaviors used, and relief behaviors justified" (p. 281). The expectations can include things such as beliefs, needs, goals, wishes, and feelings. The relief behaviors also cover psychosomatic complaints, hallucinations, delusions, sexual activity, risk-taking behavior, denial, intellectualizing, drug use, humor, self-reflection, discussion with others, validation, and problem-solving to seek the sources of difficulty. These are only a few of the relief behaviors that can be used.

People (not just clients) generally develop patterns of relief behaviors that they tend to use over and over again. Obviously, some of these patterns are more helpful than others. Anxiety is often a basis for the client to seek assistance from the nurse. At times, problems created through these relief behaviors bring the client to seek the services of the nurse. At other times, the client seeks assistance because they find the relief behaviors inadequate in relieving the anxiety.

Peplau (1989a) describes how the nurse can assist the client to channel anxiety productively. First, the client needs to be aware of and be able to name the anxiety. Then, the client needs to see the connection between the anxiety and the relief behavior. Finally, the client formulates and states expectations. This final part of the process includes an understanding of the connection between held expectations and what actually happened, and consideration of factors amenable to control. Working through this process usually takes place over time and during several interactions. The author has had some experiences with clients who have chronic mental health conditions where it has taken months for the client to even be aware of the anxiety and to name it.

Anxiety has been described by Peplau as existing along a continuum including mild, moderate, severe, and panic. Although it is possible to experience a state of no anxiety (euphoria), this seldom occurs. As human beings, we constantly face a barrage of information and other stimuli that pose at least some minor threat to our self-views. Therefore, in most nurse–client encounters, both the nurse and client will be experiencing some anxiety.

As a person's anxiety increases, that person's focus of attention becomes narrower. At the lower end of the anxiety continuum, anxiety may actually be useful in assisting the person to focus on important details. A common example would be writing an exam without being aware of other people or distractions in the room. At higher levels of anxiety, the focus of attention may become so narrow that the individual only sees small details without being able to see the larger picture. A similar example would be the student who becomes so concerned about one exam item that the total time is spent on that item and the exam is not completed. For similar reasons, problem-solving may be enhanced at lower levels of anxiety but inhibited as anxiety increases. The nurse and client need to monitor anxiety levels and attempt to keep anxiety at mild to moderate levels.

Peplau (1973b) describes how the nursing approach must consider the current anxiety level of the client. For example, as the client's anxiety is increased, the nurse would need to use increasingly short, concrete sentences to be understood. At the severe or panic levels, it would be inappropriate to use sentences with more than two or three words. It may be that even short sentences will not be understood by the client in panic, and the nurse will need to use presence as a simple non-verbal communication. The nurse also needs to be aware of the impact of anxiety on the client's current problem-solving and learning abilities and adjust accordingly. Generally, at severe or panic levels of anxiety, no new learning can take place.

Anxiety can be transmitted interpersonally (Peplau, 1989a). It is for this reason that the nurse needs to monitor his or her own anxiety. The anxious nurse will communicate anxiety to the client and vice versa. A common situation where this can occur is when the client feels out of control and the nurse fears a physical threat. This situation can easily escalate to a self-fulfilling prophecy (i.e., the client loses control and becomes assaultive). Such situations can more easily be prevented by intervening with the anxiety at lower levels and not allowing one's own anxiety to escalate the situation.

Learning

Peplau has described eight stages in the learning process. These are: 1. to observe, 2. to describe, 3. to analyze, 4. to formulate, 5. to validate, 6. to test, 7. to integrate, and 8. to utilize (Peplau,

1971). Each stage in the learning process is also a competency. Therefore, as one's learning increases, so do one's competencies.

Different individuals will be at different competency levels within the stages of learning. Even within one individual, a wide degree of variation is possible. For example, a person with generally high learning abilities may have a dramatic drop in such abilities when faced with a high anxiety-producing situation.

It is important that the nurse determines the current stage of learning of the client so that appropriate comments can be made to build on the current level and to assist the client to move to the next level. For example, if the client is at the very basic level of only being able to observe but unable to share the observations, the nurse would ask simple questions related to observation. Peplau (1971) gives examples of basic questions such as, "What do you see?" and "What is that noise?" As the person responds to these questions, they begin movement to the next stage – to describe.

There is an assumption that all people will at least be able to observe on some level, even if they cannot respond. For example, with a comatose client, the nurse could use the assumption of the ability to observe. The nurse in this situation may say, "I am now going to wash your face," and recognize the client's ability for some level of observation.

Forchuk and Voorberg (1991), in a program evaluation of a community mental health program based on Peplau's theory, found that clients were able to increase their current stage of learning. For example, upon admission, 60% of the clients with chronic mental illnesses were at the first stage of learning; only 20% remained at this level after two years.

Thinking: Preconceptions and Self-Understanding

Thinking is an internal cognitive process. The thoughts of another person can only be inferred through observation of language and behavior. The concept of thinking may be particularly important for the nurse when working with clients experiencing difficulty with their thinking processes. Examples include clients with thought disorders related to chronic mental illnesses such as schizophrenia, clients with developmental disabilities, and clients with organic brain disorders or brain injuries. The section on communication describes the integral relationship between thought and language as well as appropriate approaches to assist clients with their thinking through the use of language.

Specific thinking processes of both the nurse and client will impact the evolving nurse–client relationship. These include the preconceptions that the nurse and client have of each other and the self-understanding of the nurse and client.

Preconceptions are the initial impressions the nurse and client have of each other, before they know each other. Preconceptions may be formed through stereotyping, gossip, or past experiences with persons considered similar to the partner in the new dyad. Forchuk (1992b) found that both the nurses' and clients' preconceptions of each other were highly predictive of progress in the evolving therapeutic relationship. She also found that these initial impressions were quite stable, with very little change over the first six months of the relationship. This study underlined the importance of considering both nurse and client factors: The nurse needs to be aware of preconceptions of the client, particularly negative impressions that may impede progress in the relationship. Similarly, client impressions should also be explored. If negative preconceptions cannot be worked through, a therapeutic transfer of the client to another nurse should be considered.

Self-understanding is also a specific thinking pattern that may influence the evolving relationship. Within Peplau's theory, the concept of self-understanding has an unequal importance for the nurse and client. Self-understanding is considered a critical attribute of the nurse.

Through self-reflection and supervision, the nurse needs to be constantly aware of how their own issues and behaviors are influencing the relationship. It is expected that the nurse's self-understanding will grow through therapeutic work with clients.

Clients may also experience an increase in self-understanding through the therapeutic relationship. However, an increase in interpersonal and problem-solving competencies is the client-related goal of the relationship rather than self-understanding. Self-understanding is a helpful side effect of the process of developing these competencies.

Competencies

Competencies are skills that have evolved through practice. Peplau (1973a) states that we all have numerous interpersonal and problem-solving capacities, but in order to become competencies, they must be developed over time and through practice. The nurse–client relationship provides a venue for the development of capacities into competencies. For example, learning to share selected experiences verbally may be a capacity that the client has not developed, but may be developed during the time spent with the nurse. Other examples of competencies/capacities include sitting for five minutes in the presence of another person, discussing one topic for five minutes, learning to trust, describing one's feelings to another person, identifying personal goals, and choosing a strategy to move toward a specific goal. From these examples, it can be seen that there are a wide variety of competencies and the competencies that develop will vary considerably with different client situations. The specific competencies evolve through the developing relationship.

It is expected that the nurse will also develop competencies through the evolving relationship. These would also be primarily of a problem-solving or interpersonal nature. For example, the nurse may learn how a specific person copes with hallucinations, how to remain silent for longer periods of time to allow the client the opportunity to initiate conversation, or she or he may develop increased empathy for a certain life situation. As the nurse's competencies grow, so does their ability to help other people in similar situations; however, it is the client's development of competencies, not the nurse's, that is the priority. Parallel to the nurse's development of self-understanding, the nurse's competencies develop as a beneficial side effect of the therapeutic relationship, while the client's competencies develop as a goal of the therapeutic relationship.

Although the idea that the client's competencies take priority may seem obvious, it is sometimes forgotten in practice. It often appears more expedient for the nurse to complete an activity (e.g., feeding, making a bed, setting an out-patient appointment, listing alternatives, searching out community resources, summarizing progress) rather than the client. Of course, if this occurs, the nurse develops the competency rather than the client.

Clinical Phenomena

Peplau encourages nurses to be aware of the patterns with clinical phenomena. Observing patterns in the development and resolution of specific clinical issues allows learning from one clinical situation to potentially assist in others, which now negates the uniqueness of each situation and each client. It recognizes that each person and situation, although unique, can reveal aspects of a larger pattern.

Examples of clinical concepts that Peplau has explored are loneliness and hallucinations. Concepts are defined and operationalized with the identification of critical attributes that include the observable behaviors associated with the clinical phenomena. For example, observable signs that a person is having auditory hallucinations might include talking to an unobserved person and describing hearing voices in one's head. The nurse could identify a client with such behavior as having a pattern consistent with auditory hallucinations. Such behaviors may also be consistent with other patterns, for example, the pattern of a peak religious experience. In this section, the clinical concepts of loneliness and hallucinations are very briefly described as examples of clinical phenomena.

Loneliness

Peplau describes the problem of loneliness. She defines loneliness as "an unnoticed inability to do anything while alone" (Peplau, 1989b, p. 256). Loneliness is contrasted with lonesomeness (a wish to be with others) and aloneness (being without company). She describes the development of loneliness through difficult early interpersonal relationships.

Peplau (1989b) describes the importance of the nurse being aware of clients' defenses of loneliness; examples include time-oriented complaints (endless days), relating to others in an overly familiar or anonymous manner, planlessness, or overplanning.

The nurse assists the client with loneliness by establishing a therapeutic relationship, which will include contact and limit setting. Where appropriate, the nurse and client also plan for potentially positive peer relationships.

Hallucinations

Peplau (1989a) defines hallucinations as consisting of "illusory figures, perceived *as if* they were real" (p. 312). Peplau describes the phases through which hallucinations develop in an attempt to avoid anxiety and mitigate loneliness. While hallucinations and psychosis are generally understood to have biological roots, we still do not fully understand why certain people develop certain delusions and hallucinations from the very wide range of possibilities. The experience, understanding, and labeling of hallucinations and what is considered a hallucination is strongly influenced by culture (Laroi et al., 2014).

The nurse needs to be aware that the experience of hallucinations seems very real to the client. The nurse will carefully use language that does not reinforce the existence of the hallucinations as being mutual experiences of reality. For example, the nurse might say, "What do the voices you are hearing say?" Peplau (1989a) states that the client needs to learn alternative ways of coping with anxiety and loneliness so that the hallucinations are not needed (pp. 319–324). While we have many medications to assist with hallucinations and other symptoms of psychosis, adherence to medication is often an issue. In the study in the second chapter of Peplau (1989a), some clients identified their auditory hallucination and the nurse as their only sources of social support. It is not surprising in these situations that there may be reluctance to lose the "voices" by taking medication.

In summary, Peplau has identified a wide range of concepts that impact on the practice of the nurse and the evolving nurse–client relationship. These include interpersonal factors, intrapersonal factors, and specific clinical phenomena.

2 The Orientation Phase of the Nurse–Client Relationship

Testing Peplau's Theory

Cheryl Forchuk

Hildegard Peplau described the therapeutic nurse–client relationship as the crux of nursing (Peplau 1952/1991, 1962, 1964, 1965). According to Peplau (1952/1991), the nurse–client relationship evolves through three interlocking phases: 'orientation', 'working' (subdivided into 'identification' and 'exploitation'), and 'resolution'. Despite wide use of Peplau's theory in practice, it has not been empirically tested through research. The purpose of this investigation was to test Peplau's theory regarding influences during the orientation phase of the nurse–client relationship. This report focuses only on the hypotheses-testing aspect of the investigation.

The initial phase of the therapeutic relationship has been the most predictive of outcomes in psychotherapy with individuals with chronic mental illness (Hartley & Strupp, 1983; Luborsky, 1976). Difficulty in establishing therapeutic relationships is also related to poor outcomes in treatment (Horowitz, 1974; Luborsky, 1976; Orlinsky & Howard, 1978). Frank and Gunderson (1990) studied the therapeutic alliance and treatment outcomes of 143 individuals with non-chronic schizophrenia. They found the initial six months in the alliance was a critical time period: If a 'good' alliance did not develop in this time, it was unlikely to develop at all.

Hypotheses

The hypotheses for this study focused on variables measured at the beginning of the relationship that were expected to be related to the development of the therapeutic relationship:

1. Clients' more positive preconceptions of the nurse will be related to greater progress in the development of therapeutic relationships.
2. Nurses' more positive preconceptions of the client will be related to greater progress in the development of therapeutic relationships.
3. Clients' more positive interpersonal relationships will be related to greater progress in the development of therapeutic relationships.
4. Nurses' more positive interpersonal relationships will be related to greater progress in the development of therapeutic relationships.
5. Higher levels of anxiety in the client will be related to less progress in the development of therapeutic relationships.
6. Higher levels of anxiety in the nurse will be related to less progress in the development of therapeutic relationships.
7. Taken together, the client's preconceptions of the nurse, level of anxiety, and interpersonal relationships will be a better predictor of progress in the development of therapeutic relationships than any one client variable alone.

8. Taken together, the nurse's preconceptions of the client, level of anxiety, and interpersonal relationships will be a better predictor of progress in the development of therapeutic relationships than any one nurse variable alone.

Methodology

Design

The investigation employed a prospective panel longitudinal design. The study was correlational and used the initial results for developing the independent variables (preconceptions, interpersonal relationships, and anxiety) to predict later results for the dependent variable (development of the therapeutic relationship). Data collection periods took place at zero months (time-1), three months (time-2), and six months (time-3) into the nurse–client relationship.

Instruments

Development of the Therapeutic Relationship

Development of the therapeutic relationship was measured with two instruments. These instruments were the Relationship Form (Forchuk & Brown, 1989) and the Working Alliance Inventory (Horvath & Greenberg, 1986, 1989).

The Relationship Form specifies nurse and client behaviors at each phase of the nurse–client relationship. Forchuk and Brown (1989) found the inter-rater reliability within one point to be 91%, and where disagreement existed, a clinical nurse specialist consistently rated the relationship one point higher than the nurse in the relationship. For the current study, the nurse in the relationship validated the determination of the duration of the orientation phase with a clinical nurse specialist, who was blind to other measures.

The Working Alliance Inventory (WAI) is a 36-item, self-report instrument with parallel forms for clients and therapists. It examined nurses' and clients' perception of the bond, tasks, and goals within the evolving therapeutic relationship. It was administered at time-2 (three months) and time-3 (six months) since it requires that the therapist and client have been working together for at least two months. For this investigation, the Cronbach's alpha was 0.93 for the client form and 0.95 for the therapist form. The number of weeks spent in orientation on the Relationship Form was significantly related to both the WAI therapist form ($r = -0.41$) and client form ($r = -0.36$).

Preconceptions

Preconceptions of nurses and clients were measured through semantic differential scales (Osgood et al., 1957). These scales are attitude measuring instruments with 7-point scales between bipolar adjective pairs (e.g., good–bad). The specific adjective pairs used were determined through a preliminary survey of 20 newly formed nurse–client dyads who were asked to give descriptions of each other through comparisons with descriptions of nurse and client stereotypes described in the literature. Cronbach's alpha for the various time intervals, including both client and nurse forms, ranged from 0.75 to 0.86.

Other Interpersonal Relationships

Other interpersonal relationships were measured through the Personal Resource Questionnaire (PRQ; Brandt & Weinert, 1981). The PRQ is a two-part, self-report instrument designed to measure characteristics of social support. For this investigation, only Part Two was used. Part Two measures the quality of interpersonal relationships (social integration, intimacy, worth, nurturance, and assistance) through 25 items with Likert scales. Cronbach's alpha for the various time intervals, including both client and nurse results, ranged from 0.87 to 0.94.

Anxiety

Anxiety was measured through the Beck Anxiety Inventory (BAI; Beck et al., 1988). The BAI is a 21-item, self-report scale that has been developed for measuring the severity of anxiety in psychiatric populations. Cronbach's alpha for the various time intervals, including both client and nurse results, ranged from 0.68 to 0.91. The only alpha below 0.85 was the nurse result of 0.68 at time-2, which reflected a greater diversity of responses at that interval.

Sample

The investigation utilized non-probability, purposive sampling of 124 newly formed nurse–client dyads. Potential dyads were identified within selected long-term programmes serving the chronically mentally ill population within south central Ontario, Canada. The rights, dignity, and anonymity of all subjects were protected throughout the study.

Of the 124 dyads included in time-1, 57 dyads were included at time-2 and 38 dyads at time-3. The reasons dyads were not included at time-2 and/or time-3 were: clients' discharge (45 for time-2, eight for time-3); transfer or leave of client or nurse (12 for time-2, seven for time-3); nurse or client declining further participation in study (nine for time-2, three for time-3), and client death (one for time-2, one for time-3). Early discharge would be generally indicative of improved functioning and within this Canadian sample, would be unrelated to healthcare insurance.

Sample Characteristics

Although 124 dyads were in the sample, some nurses were involved in more than one dyad. A total of 74 different nurses participated. Within the 124 dyads, 107 were registered nurses (including all of the community nurses), and 17 were registered nursing assistants (similar to the American licensed practical nurse); 119 were female, and five were male. The average age was 39.7 years with 16.9 years in nursing.

Of the 124 initial clients, 83 were male, 41 were female. Psychiatric diagnoses were available on only 81 clients: schizophrenia (n=57), affective disorder (n=10), schizoaffective disorder (n=4), personality disorder (n=4), and other psychiatric diagnoses (n=6). The average age was 44.1, with 6.4 previous psychiatric admissions. The average duration of the most recent psychiatric hospitalization was 35.8 months. The initial sample included 95 hospitalized clients and 29 in transitional or community programmes.

Results

The Relationship Form was completed on 94 dyads: 51 who completed orientation, 30 who discontinued the relationship while still in the orientation phase, and 13 who remained in orientation after six months. In calculations involving the number of weeks in orientation, only the 51 dyads who completed orientation are included. See Table 2.1 for a summary of results of primary hypotheses.

Single Variables and the Therapeutic Relationship

The results for the first six hypotheses are reported in Table 2.1. From this table, it can be seen that the preconceptions of both the nurse and client were most strongly related to the development of the therapeutic relationship on either measure. Clients' other relationships were significant on the WAI only and nurses' other interpersonal relationships were not significant. Anxiety of nurses and clients was not significantly related to progress in the relationship.

Combined Variables and the Therapeutic Relationship

The seventh and eighth hypotheses suggest the explanatory power of the combination of client or nurse variables will be greater than single client or nurse variables. Two multiple regressions were calculated for each of these hypotheses. One analysis used the number of weeks in orientation and the other the development of the therapeutic alliance (WAI at time-2) as indicators of progress in the relationship.

For the seventh hypothesis (using weeks in orientation as the dependent measure), only the client's preconceptions of the nurse were significantly predictive. The multiple R of 0.42 (R^2, 0.17) was only slightly greater than the simple r(0.37) for preconceptions. In using client scores on the WAI as the dependent measure, the client's interpersonal relationships and preconceptions were both predictive. The multiple R was 0.58 (R^2 0.34) compared to the simple rs of 0.47 for interpersonal relationships and –0.38 for preconceptions. Therefore, the seventh hypothesis was partially supported.

For the eighth hypothesis (using weeks in orientation as the dependent measure) the nurse's preconceptions of the client were the most predictive variable, but this was not statistically significant. The multiple R of 0.37 (R^2, 0.14) was only slightly greater than the simple r of 0.30 for preconceptions. The variable of preconceptions was the only predictive variable when using the WAI as the indicator of progress in the relationship. The multiple R of 0.66 was a negligible change over the simple r of 0.65 for preconceptions. Therefore, the eighth hypothesis was not supported.

A regression analysis including both nurse and client variables identified in the hypotheses was also completed. As reported in Table 2.2 (with both measures of progress in the therapeutic relationship), the R^2 values for the combination of nurse and client variables were significantly greater than when only client or only nurse variables were included.

Table 2.1 Summary of Results of Primary Hypotheses

Independent Variables	*r*	
	Weeks in Orientation	*Working Alliance Inventory (WAI)*
Client preconceptions	0.37*	−0.38*
Nurse preconceptions	0.31*	−0.69*
Client interpersonal relationships	−0.17	0.48*
Nurse interpersonal relationships	−0.05	0.00
Client anxiety	0.01	0.09
Nurse anxiety	0.22	−0.08

*$p \leq 0.05$, hypothesis supported.

Forchuk, C. (1994). The orientation phase of the nurse-client relationship: Testing Peplau's theory. *Journal of Advanced Nursing*, 20, 532–537. https://doi.org/10.1111/j.1365-2648.1994.tb02392.x

Table 2.2 Combined Nurse and Client Variables

Variables	R^2
Weeks in orientation	
Nurse variables	0.14
Client variables	0.17
Combined variables	0.38
Working Alliance Inventory	
Nurse variables	0.44
Client variables	0.34
Combined variables	0.61

Forchuk, C. (1994). The orientation phase of the nurse-client relationship: Testing Peplau's theory. *Journal of Advanced Nursing, 20*, 532–537. https://doi.org/10.1111/j.1365-2648.1994.tb02392.x

Discussion

The findings of this study support some of the tenets of Peplau's theory, but not others. This has implications for further theory development or refinement, research, and practice.

The concept of preconceptions and its relative importance in the evolving therapeutic relationship received considerable support through the findings of this investigation. The support for the first two hypotheses related to nurse and client preconceptions corroborates some of the most essential propositions of Peplau's theory.

The finding that both the nurses' and clients' preconceptions were significant is supportive of an interpersonal approach. Peplau's theory recognizes that the nurse must use awareness of self and self-reflection as vigilantly as assessment of the client situation.

The findings may suggest that the interpersonal relationships of the client are important but not those of the nurse. In this study, only clients reported poor relationships with others. The lowest rating by a nurse was neutral.

Viewing a specific relationship may be quite different from viewing the totality of relationships. For example, within a totality of generally positive relationships, the nurse (or client) may have had specific negative experiences with clients (or nurses) perceived to be similar to the current client (or nurse). It may therefore be prudent to first test the influence of a narrower range of other interpersonal relationships before disregarding nurses' other relationships.

Anxiety

The anxiety scores of both nurses and clients were not significant to the evolving relationship in this study. In Peplau's theory, anxiety is discussed within many contexts (Peplau, 1973b, 1989a). Anxiety would be expected to develop at varying levels within the specific nurse–client relationship, but would also be expected to occur at other times, independent of the nurse–client relationship. If further study found no support for even a narrower context of anxiety, the theory would need to de-emphasize the relative importance of anxiety.

Thoughts and Feelings Towards Clients

The findings suggest that nurses need to be aware of their thoughts and feelings towards their clients. Both negative and positive preconceptions seem to form very early in the relationship and undergo very little change. Yet, they have a significant relationship to the duration of the orientation phase.

Discharge of Clients Still in the Orientation Phase

The number of clients discharged or transferred while still in the orientation phase may raise clinical concerns. This happened only with hospitalized clients. The 30 clients discontinued represented almost one in three (of 95) of all hospitalized clients in the study. This implies that this large group of clients were discharged or transferred without establishing trust with their nurses or identifying problems to be worked on during hospitalization.

Limitations

Potential threats to the internal validity of the study include threats due to multiple testing, evaluation apprehension, the use of multiple sites, and that the process of asking questions related to the relationship may change it.

Mortality was a potential threat to external validity. Another threat was that the sample of subjects completing orientation (n=51) was less than the minimum number suggested by power analysis (n=83) to adequately test the hypotheses. This increased the risk of type two error, that is, the risk of rejecting a true hypothesis.

Conclusion

A stated purpose for this investigation was the testing of an established nursing theory. This is essential since such theories are seldom tested (Silva, 1986). This investigation tested Peplau's theory by determining if variables identified within her theory as significant were related to the development of the nurse–client relationship. Preconceptions of both the client and nurse were related to the development of the therapeutic relationship. These preconceptions developed very early in the relationship and underwent almost no change over a six month period. There was support for the importance of other relationships for clients but not for nurses. Anxiety was not found to be significantly related to the time in the orientation phase. The investigation therefore supports some tenets of Peplau's theory, but not others. This gives direction for future research and theory refinement. Specifically, the importance of anxiety and other relationships may be less important than the theory currently suggests. Continued testing of nursing theory will guide both future theory refinement and the application of theory in practice.

Acknowledgment

The author would like to acknowledge the assistance of her doctoral committee chair, Laurel Northouse, RN, PhD. During the completion of this research the author was a Fellow of the Ontario Ministry of Health, Health Research Personnel Development Program, and the recipient of the Baxter Fellowship in Nursing Science, Canadian Nurses Foundation.

Part II

Care Recipient Perspectives

This section will introduce the reader to what care recipients find promotes the building of therapeutic relationships. Therapeutic relationships include a partnership between the person coming for help and the person providing help. The purpose of the therapeutic relationship is to assist the person receiving care. We need to consider the uniqueness of each person and to consider our own understanding of the perspective of the care recipient.

The set of papers will lay out what people may perceive as unhelpful approaches. Oftentimes, the perceptions surrounding the deterioration of the relationship appears early, but these signs may not be easily recognized by the nurse or other care providers.

Chapter 3 is "A Review of Our Understanding of the Care Recipient Perspective" written by Sebastian Gyamfi and Shirley Tran. This chapter reviews current research on the therapeutic relationship from the perspective of the care recipient. In particular, what do people find helpful and not helpful as the relationship develops? It is interesting to note the consistency across time, countries, and care contexts about what is truly important.

Chapter 4 is a reprint of a qualitative "test" of Peplau's theory from the care recipient perspective. The chapter is entitled "Factors Influencing Movement of Chronic Psychiatric Patients from the Orientation to the Working Phase of the Nurse–Client Relationship on an Inpatient Unit" and is written by Cheryl Forchuk, Jan Westwell, Mary-Lou Martin, Wendy Azzopardi, Donna Kosterewa-Tolman, and Margaret Hux [previously published as Forchuk, C., Westwell, J., Martin, M.-L., Bamber-Azzapardi[1], W., Kosterewa-Tolman, D., & Hux, M. (1998). Factors influencing movement of chronic psychiatric patients from the orientation to the working phase of the nurse-client relationship on an inpatient unit. *Perspectives in Psychiatric Care*, *34*(1), 36–44. https://doi.org/10.1111/j.1744-6163.1998.tb00998.x]. This chapter summarizes a qualitative study involving interviews with care recipients and nurses during the evolution of therapeutic and non-therapeutic relationships. Videotapes of nurse–client interactions also informed the study. This chapter highlights care recipient interviews and their understanding of the evolving relationship.

Note

1 Previous publication misspelled Azzopardi.

3 A Review of Our Understanding of the Care Recipient Perspective

Sebastian Gyamfi and Shirley Tran

The relationship between the client and care provider ('provider') constitutes one of the key dynamics in the therapeutic outcomes of every client (Ardito & Rabellino, 2011; Norcross & Lambert, 2018; Nurses' Association of New Brunswick [NANB], 2015; Peplau, 1991; Schottenfeld et al., 2016). Therapeutic relationships are vital due to their ability to positively impact change among clients compared to the treatment itself (Ardito & Rabellino, 2011; Easterbrook & Meehan, 2017) and require efforts by all stakeholders (i.e., clients, family, caregivers, and policymakers). Therapeutic relationships are grounded in purposeful, goal-directed interpersonal relational processes that are directed at advancing the best interests and outcomes for the client. They constitute a key dimension of treatment and all subsequent client–provider interactions. The therapeutic relationship can be conceptualized as follows:

> A [therapeutic relationship] is a human-to-human interaction that usually take place between a client (patient) and a care giver (therapist) in or outside a health setting (e.g., hospital, clinic) aimed at helping the client in recovery. It is a goal-based and problem solving relationship – Identifying strengths and weaknesses, finding ways of meeting client needs, and promoting adaptive growth in the client.
>
> (Gyamfi, 2016, p. 38)

The therapeutic relationship is also conceptualized as an interactive relationship with the client and family that is associated with positive caring and clear boundaries of professional behaviour (Ridling et al., 2011).

Burgeoning recovery models of care encourage individuals to be resilient and stay in control of their life, even without full remission of their symptoms (Jacob, 2015). Therapeutic relationships assist clients to look beyond the limitations that may be imposed by unresolved symptoms (Kornhaber et al., 2016) and help people achieve their goals, aspirations, and dreams. Clients' willingness to actively participate in care depends heavily on the level of interpersonal interaction that occurs between the caregiver and the recipient (Chichirez & Purcărea, 2018; Kornhaber et al., 2016).

Therapeutic relationships ought to protect the client's dignity, autonomy, and privacy and allow for the development of trust and respect. The NANB (2015) believes that an effective therapeutic relationship should be planned, time-limited, and goal-directed. The therapeutic relationship is a fundamental factor of psychological therapy. Helpful relationships between clients and providers strongly predict positive care outcomes (Easterbrook & Meehan, 2017; Kornhaber et al., 2016). Involvement of family in the care process has increased over the last ten years due to the vital role that families play in the life of the client (see Doser & Norup, 2016; Guldager et al., 2019). Therefore, this review sheds light on the perspective of clients and family in relation to the attitudes and behaviours of the care provider.

Clients' Perceptions About Care Providers' Attitudes and Behaviours

In contemporary times, various research reports indicate that individuals receiving care are more likely to establish good therapeutic relationships when they encounter healthcare professionals who have good interpersonal and communication skills (Knobloch-Fedders, 2008). Clients are more likely to form good relationships with providers when care providers are open, flexible, and honest about the support they are willing to provide. The providers' ability to communicate and demonstrate empathy and understanding to clients has been found to boost the therapeutic relationship (Knobloch-Fedders, 2008). Specifically, seeking ideas from clients about the goals and methods of treatment before implementation has the capacity of fostering collaboration during the client–provider interaction process.

Recently, Norcross and Lambert (2018) completed a review of 16 meta-analyses that evaluated the evidence on particular elements of the therapeutic relationship and associated client treatment outcomes. The authors found that certain relationship factors, such as agreement on therapy goals, collecting client feedback throughout the course of treatment, and repairing ruptures in the therapeutic alliance, had significant but small to medium effects on therapeutic outcomes for clients. The problems that may arise in the course of the interaction are as vital as the positive outcomes that may be observed using other interventions, such as physical treatment modalities. Norcross and Lambert (2018) affirmed that effects of 'other treatment methods' and the therapeutic relationship are inseparable and in constant, complex, and reciprocal interaction, shaping and informing each other in the context in which the relationship and treatment are applied.

Norcross and Lambert's (2018) meta-analysis affirmed that creating a therapeutic relationship with the client should be a fundamental goal of every provider, even before other treatments commence. Providers should engage in ongoing assessment of existing relational activities, such as alliances, empathy, and interrelation or cohesion, for appropriate and timely responses towards more positive client outcomes. Positive client outcomes can be achieved by the provider being aware of and tailoring care towards the 'individuality' of the client in relation to their cultural identity and needs. The analysis uncovered that providers who demonstrate cultural humility and track clients' satisfaction with cultural responsiveness were more likely to enhance client engagement and retention, as well as increase treatment success.

The Norcross and Lambert (2018) review revealed the need for providers to ensure routine monitoring of client satisfaction to ascertain comfort. Such monitoring efforts were likely to create increased opportunities for the providers to re-establish collaboration efforts, improve or modify the relationship, and adjust unhelpful treatment procedures that may be hindering care outcomes, especially for clients who were at risk of relationship deterioration. The authors categorized their findings into elements that worked or did not work. They found good alliance (individual, couple, and family), collaboration, goal consensus, cohesion in group therapy, empathy, positive regard, and affirmation to be effective (i.e., 'what works'), while poor alliances, poor cohesion in group therapy, and lack of empathy, cohesion, consensus, and positive regard to be ineffective (i.e., 'what does not work'). The collection and delivery of client feedback was classified as 'demonstrably effective' due to the high numbers of sufficient studies about these concepts.

In another meta-analytic review of 82 studies, Elliott and colleagues (2018) examined relationships between provider empathy and patient success at the end of treatment. Analysis revealed that clients with more empathic therapists tend to be happier, healthier, and experience more progress in treatment, which culminates into greater improvement at the end of the day.

In the United Kingdom, Sweeney et al. (2014) examined the relationship between therapeutic alliance and service user satisfaction in mental health inpatient wards and crisis house alternatives. They studied 384 service users and 13 staff in a cross-sectional mixed-methods design. Service users were found to value relationships with staff who demonstrated kindness, warmth, empathy, honesty, trustworthiness, reassurance, friendliness, helpfulness, calmness, and humour. The service users also revealed that crisis house environments felt homely, relaxed, and peaceful and made them feel like the space/environment was shared with staff, leading to a positive atmosphere on the ward. The staff affirmed that lessening restrictions on liberty of service users (i.e., in crisis houses) reduced anger, frustration, and aggression, resulting in a less volatile and hostile ward environment. The care providers again added that when staff appeared engaged with and interested in service users through simple acts, such as asking about one's day, it had important implications on their morale and relationships; this made service users feel motivated, giving them a reason for being in hospital. In all of these demands and efforts by providers, Sweeney and colleagues suggested that staff needed support from management to maintain the motivation of meeting job demands, while being able to communicate effectively with service users.

Findings from Moreno-Poyato and colleagues' (2016) narrative review of 48 articles in relation to nurses' and clients' perspectives of the therapeutic relationship in the context of inpatient psychiatric care were similar to those found two years earlier by Sweeney et al. (2014) in the UK. Moreno-Poyato et al. (2016) found that clients expected certain qualities of their caregivers, particularly acceptance and respect (i.e., absence of prejudice). They also identified that clients valued empathic understanding, listening, authenticity, honesty, and trustworthiness as helpful factors by nurses. Other dynamics, such as nurses being accessible to the client, demonstrating companionship and friendliness, and having a sense of humor, presented a perception of mutual respect among the clients, which ultimately aided the therapeutic relationship.

Bolsinger et al. (2020) also performed a narrative review of 49 articles and found that desirable staff attitudes and behaviors were vital in ensuring fruitful relationships during therapy. For instance, dialogue between clients and their providers on delicate subjects, such as coercion, were useful and very much desired by clients. Similar to the findings in Moreno-Poyato et al. (2016), the recent study by Bolsinger and colleagues (2020) also emphasized the need for staff to understand clients' needs in order to meet them accordingly, which could be identified by establishing transparent communication on delicate topics. Transparent communication may diminish misunderstandings between clients and staff, especially among involuntary admissions.

Globally, Bolsinger and colleagues' (2020) review provides insight into why there is a need for providers to collaborate with clients and their close relatives. For example, Bolsinger et al. (2020) found that providers' involvement of clients in the process of decision-making, wherever possible, contributed to or predicted positive therapeutic outcomes, including medication adherence and decreasing clients' perceptions of coercion. In the context of psychiatric emergency, the Bolsinger-led narrative review found that establishing crisis intervention teams to visit clients in their home suggests overall positive perceptions about the provider–client relationship. They believed that home-based interventions may also enable family and other social contacts to be better accounted for in the therapeutic process.

Client-Family–Provider Relationships

Therapeutic relationship models over the years have centered mostly on the client–provider relationship. Emerging literature demonstrates the need for involving both the client and their family in the therapeutic care process.

The involvement of a client's family becomes particularly important in situations where client communication and decision-making are hampered (Guldager et al., 2019). Experts have established that involving family can give clients a voice and a proxy to advocate for clients in times of crucial need (Doser & Norup, 2016; Guldager et al., 2019). Families can also act as experts in providing vital information that would otherwise elude care professionals (Guldager et al., 2019). For example, family members can describe the usual characteristics and behaviours of the client, which can be helpful to inform providers on clinical progress and outcomes of treatment or whether the client requires additional intervention. Focusing care on establishing a trusting relationship with the client and their family at the beginning of hospitalization had the potential of promoting involvement in the rehabilitation process through tailored support, regardless of the individual's personal resources or position in society (Guldager et al., 2019).

Support of treatment by including the client's family is associated with successful therapeutic relationships and care outcomes (Knobloch-Fedders, 2008; Kornhaber et al., 2016; McGinnis et al., 2013). McGinnis et al. (2013) emphasized family engagement during client care to promote better therapeutic care outcomes. The researchers described the client and family as a learning healthcare system and therefore focusing care modalities on both clients and their families has the potential to influence clinical, health, and economic outcomes in several ways. For instance, clients and their families are able to bring their personal knowledge forward regarding the suitability of some treatment modalities for a particular client's circumstances and preferences.

What Do Clients Perceive as Unhelpful in Establishing a Good Therapeutic Relationship?

The quality of the therapeutic relationship is vital to treatment outcomes irrespective of the type of treatment being given to the client (Knobloch-Fedders, 2008). For instance, establishing positive and trusting relationships during the care process constitutes a vital component for enhancing the effectiveness of care and subsequent outcomes (Feo et al., 2017); however, there are attitudes and behaviors among providers that some clients perceive as not helpful for successful care outcomes.

For instance, Norcross and Lambert (2018) identified poor therapeutic alliance with the client, low levels of cohesion during group therapy, poor collaboration, poor consensus building, lack of empathy, and non-existing positive regard as unhelpful attitudes and behaviours among providers. Being non-receptive to providing clients with feedback on treatment progress, ignoring therapeutic alliance ruptures, and lacking awareness of countertransference was also unhelpful. Regarding the client as a consumer and providing untrustworthy treatment amidst flat emotional attitudes and behaviours can also influence treatment dropout or treatment failure. Unhealthy client–provider relationships can yield negative consequences for the client and may violate care protocols, boundaries, and ethical standards of acceptable behaviour, or even cause significant harm to the client and family.

Theodoridou and colleagues (2012) studied perceived coercion within the therapeutic relationship among 116 clients with psychiatric diagnoses. They found that perceived coercion by clients led to higher levels of symptoms and perceived loss of autonomy, which led care recipients to rate the therapeutic relationship negatively. Similarly, Soto et al. (2019) observed that providers confronting clients, demonstrating inflexibility, or displaying egocentricity obstructed the client–provider relationship. They further commented that providers being culturally arrogant and disregarding the client's cultural beliefs by imposing their own beliefs (e.g., in relation to gender, racial/ethnic perspectives, sexual orientation, and other preferences onto the client) were detrimental to care outcomes.

In their 2016 narrative review, Moreno-Poyato and colleagues found that providers' limited accessibility to clients, lack of communication, intimidation, insecurity, and perceived tension in the relationship negatively affected client outcomes. Other aspects of the review revealed that when providers demonstrated a distant and unapproachable attitude, clients began to feel like they had very few chances to work together, which was particularly felt when clients believed their contributions were not included in care planning. Negative attitudes towards clients by providers can instill dehumanizing feelings, frustration, and increase clients' vulnerability to other extraneous influences that may interfere with their recovery and care outcomes.

Similarly, Bolsinger et al. (2020) found that increasing severity of symptoms in clients decreases their quality ratings of the therapeutic relationship. The review also revealed that loss of autonomy, such as in restrictive practices (e.g., closed doors, limited access for visitors, limited permissions to leave the ward, perceived coercion in relation to forcing one to take medications, physical or chemical restraints, and seclusion without consent), negatively impacted the therapeutic relationship. A lack of openness and transparency in a trustful relationship between the client and provider, such as withholding or disclosing information (e.g., death of a relative, spouse's wish to divorce), was likely to provoke aggression in acutely agitated clients. In essence, the therapeutic relationship is likely to be affected negatively when clients disagree with providers' judgements and decisions – even when providers make treatment decisions that they believe to be in the best interest of the client and are based on professional judgement. The presence of conflict among multidisciplinary teams and other clients can cause 'spill-over' effects that impact other therapeutic relationships, which are also non-therapeutic. The Bolsinger et al. (2020) study revealed that issues relating to the individuality of clients, for example, providers being oblivious to clients' culture and preferences (e.g., gender, background, ethnicity, personality, communication style, or language) were also detrimental.

In another vein, Sibeoni et al. (2020) studied factors that impede alliances in treatment among 41 persons in France. The researchers identified that maintaining appropriate boundaries or space between the client and provider influenced the care process and outcomes. Being too close or too distant from the client interfered with therapy. Again, providers controlling and constraining their clients and/or the family negatively affected care relationships and outcomes.

Conclusion

An effective therapeutic relationship helps restore and promote the health of persons receiving therapy. The inherent power differential that exists between the client and provider in the therapeutic relationship and the value of client perceptions in relationship outcomes makes it worthwhile to consider client perspectives in every care situation, be it biomedical, psychological, or social. To be successful, the therapeutic relationship ought to be regarded as a long-term bond that occurs between the client and provider. In situations where the client or family feels the absence of choice in treatment decisions, an asymmetrical, non-therapeutic relationship develops, which could result in tension and non-adherence to treatment. Decision-making that espouses client autonomy and actively includes the client and their family is therefore valuable. Findings from the studies reviewed in this chapter appear to corroborate each other, revealing that clients are more likely to bring unique and vital perspectives into their own care when the relationship is open, client-driven, and highly coordinated by the care professional (McGinnis et al., 2013). In all, client-driven care encourages the client to maintain and adhere to treatment regimens so as to foster early recovery, implying immediate need for putting in place appropriate emancipatory care protocols that are embedded in shared decision-making practices in and out of the hospital.

4 Factors Influencing Movement of Chronic Psychiatric Patients from the Orientation to the Working Phase of the Nurse–Client Relationship on an Inpatient Unit

Cheryl Forchuk, Jan Westwell, Mary-Lou Martin, Wendy Azzopardi, Donna Kosterewa-Tolman, and Margaret Hux

Hildegard Peplau's classic book, *Interpersonal Relations in Nursing*, published in 1952 and reprinted in 1991, focused on the nurse–client relationship. The work was based on the analysis of interactions of psychiatric nurse–patient dyads through process recordings and direct observations. This interpersonal focus and method were consistent with symbolic interaction theory (Mead, 1934).

According to Peplau's (1952/1991) theory, each therapeutic relationship begins with an orientation phase. In this phase, the client seeks help and tests the parameters of the relationship. The orientation phase ends when the client participates in the identification of problems and subproblems (Peplau, 1952/1988a/1991). A prolonged orientation phase can be frustrating to both nurses and clients, since any work on client problems cannot begin until this phase is completed (Forchuk & Brown, 1989; Peplau, 1996). The current study was undertaken to determine what factors help or hinder movement from the orientation phase to the working phase and what constitutes the working phase of the therapeutic relationship from the clients' perspective.

Methods

The investigation had a naturalistic qualitative design and employed an interpersonal method (see also Heifner, 1997). The interpersonal method draws upon the work of Peplau (1991) and symbolic interaction (Mead, 1934). Leininger's (1985) ethnonursing method of analyzing data was used. The focus of inquiry was the orientation phase of the nurse–client relationship as defined by Peplau (1952/1988a/1991). This period begins when the nurse and client first meet and ends when the client begins to identify problems to explore with the nurse. This report focuses on client perceptions. The study was approved through the hospital research and ethics committee and the hospital nursing research committee. The method involved a clinical nurse specialist/investigator who interviewed (a) clients diagnosed with chronic mental illnesses, and (b) inpatient nurses who had been newly assigned to these clients. All interviews were audiotaped. In addition, two videotaped nurse–client interactions were completed for each dyad. Sessions were videotaped at the beginning of the orientation phase and at the working phase.

Sample

The sample included ten newly formed nurse–client dyads on three inpatient units at a tertiary care psychiatric hospital in Southern Ontario, Canada. All nurses were registered with a minimum of ten years' psychiatric nursing experience. Eight nurses were female and two were male. Clients included six males and four females. Both dyads with a male nurse included a male client. Four clients were from admission units and six were from long-term care areas. Seven clients were diagnosed with schizophrenia and three clients were diagnosed with a major mood disorder. Nurses and clients typically met three to five times per week. Clients and nurses agreed to participate in the study and understood the purpose was to examine their evolving relationship.

Data Collection

Data were collected via audiotaped interviews with clients. The interviews were unstructured and employed broad open-ended questions related to the evolving nurse–client relationship. Examples included, "Tell me what's happening in the relationship now," and "Have you noticed anything different about your relationship lately?" The dyad was seen to have moved out of the orientation phase when the client, nurse, and clinical nurse specialist agreed that the dyad had a working relationship. In all cases, a three-way consensus existed. Clients were interviewed from two to nine times each, reflecting differences in the duration of the orientation phases.

Research Questions

In considering the move from the orientation phase to the working phase of the nurse–client relationship, the research questions were:

1. What seems to help the movement from the orientation to working phase?
2. What seems to hamper movement from the orientation to the working phase?
3. What is the nature of the therapeutic relationship in the working phase?

Data Analysis

Leininger's (1985) process of qualitative analysis was employed. This process includes:

1. Identify and list descriptors of observations and experiences of domain under study.
2. Combine raw data and descriptors into meaningful sequential units, known as patterns.
3. Identify mini patterns and determine how they relate to larger patterns.
4. Synthesize several patterns to obtain broad, comprehensive, and holistic themes.
5. Formulate theme statements to test or reaffirm phenomena. (Themes are tested/reaffirmed by reviewing against raw data and/or review of the themes with the study participants.)
6. Use confirmed themes to develop hypotheses, make decisions, and plan interventions (summarized from Leininger, 1985).

Data were transcribed verbatim, omitting names and identifying information. The three clinical nurse specialists reviewed all transcripts and developed the themes through consensus. The final phase of analysis involved a cross-comparison of themes and descriptions arising from the three data sets (client interviews, nurse interviews, and videotapes).

Results

Of the ten dyads, seven were able to establish a working relationship during the client hospital stay. The time required to do this ranged from 2.5 weeks to six months. Two dyads did not reach a working relationship and continued in the orientation phase for almost one year before switching the nurse assignment. One client was discharged after six months without establishing a working relationship. Of the three dyads not reaching the working phase, two included female nurses and one included a male nurse; two clients were male, and one was female. This essentially reflects the gender ratios in the sample.

Factors That Helped Movement from Orientation to Working Phase

Clients consistently described the importance of the planned therapeutic interaction meeting, events occurring outside of the formal meeting (e.g., on the unit), and the personal characteristics of the nurse (see Figure 4.1). Progress in the developing relationship was signified by the transition between hardly knowing the nurse to being able to identify mutual trust and understanding, and a growing confidence in the nurse. By sharing and mutually identifying problems, the partners moved toward the establishment of mutual goals. The clients found themselves willing to talk more as the relationship progressed. They described the nurse and client "getting used to" each other and "growth" as moving to a "different level" that no longer left them feeling awkward.

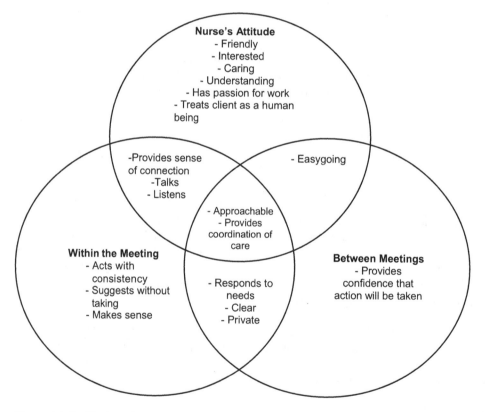

Figure 4.1 Facilitation of the Therapeutic Relationship. Forchuk, C., Westwell, J., Martin, M.-L., Bamber-Azzapardi, W., Kosterewa-Tolman, D., & Hux, M. (1998). Factors influencing movement of chronic psychiatric patients from the orientation to the working phase of the nurse-client relationship on an inpatient unit. *Perspectives in Psychiatric Care, 34*(1), 36–44. https://doi.org/10.1111/j.1744-6163.1998.tb00998.x.

Within Formal Sessions

Issues that were identified included the opportunity to talk to and be listened to, and the consistency of meeting with the same nurse over time. Descriptions of the meetings from clients include: "She seems to always be there," and "Sometimes it's [the things we talk about are] repetitive and staff tunes out. They don't hear anymore. But [my nurse] continues to listen. That's the difference." Other comments from clients regarding the nurse–client meetings included: "She listens to me, what I say. When I talk, she doesn't make a sound," "She's wonderful…and quite consistent," "She went as far as she could to help me understand…," and "She's quite unobtrusive. I don't feel she's hovering over me."

Between Formal Sessions

Clients found it important that their nurses followed through on whatever had been agreed to, such as referrals, arranging day passes, or passing along information. Following the formal meetings, clients expressed confidence that action would be taken on topics that they had discussed and that care would be coordinated with other staff, with specific attention to their needs. For example, clients said: "When I needed something, even something like going to the dentist, it happened fast."

Attitude of the Nurses

Another helping factor consistently identified was the nurse's attitude. Clients described the importance of the nurse being friendly, trusting, interested, genuine, easygoing, offering suggestions without taking control, and understanding. Helpful nurses were described as having "a passion" for their work, "treating [clients] as human beings," and "believing in me."

In summary, availability, consistency, and trust in the nurse were perceived to be important factors moving relationships from the orientation to the working phase.

Factors That Hampered Movement from Orientation to Working Phase

Several factors were identified by clients as hampering their relationships with their nurses. The unavailability of the nurse was cited most frequently, but some clients also discussed their own unavailability. Perceived inequities and distance between the nurse and client, as well as differences in realities and values, were also seen as barriers. Once these barriers developed, dyads entered into a phase of mutual withdrawal and avoidance.

Lack of Availability

One factor identified as hampering movement into the working phase was the unavailability of the primary nurse in a literal sense (e.g., through vacation, days off, or a change in assignment). At times, the relationship was hampered even when the primary nurse was available through limited, or superficial, contact with the client. Limited contact was described as not meeting regularly, meeting briefly, or meeting only in the hallway. Such limited contact was inconsistent with the hospital nursing care standards and occurred in this study only during difficult relationships. Examples of superficial contact described by clients included not meeting privately, confusion as to the identity of the assigned nurse, or the nurse's inability to make the effort to draw out the client, particularly when personal problems were difficult to discuss. Some clients believed their own unavailability, unrelated to the nurse, slowed the progress of the relationship. Clients' personal problems, such as recent losses and memory problems, sometimes left them feeling like they could not reach out to others or made it difficult to build from one session to the next.

Sense of Distance/Inequity

Clients expressed negative feelings about nurses when they perceived the nurses had a "superior attitude," as this caused them to feel they were not taken as persons and their concerns were not treated seriously. For example, some clients said, "I don't feel like a person," and "They don't acknowledge me. It's like being in limbo." Another client used the analogy of being "invisible."

Differences in Realities/Values

Nurses were perceived by clients as unaccepting of the client's reality when the nurses used technical terminology, such as "delusions," or accepted information that they heard about the client without getting to know the person. In some cases, the nurse was incorporated into the client's belief system. For example, one client believed the nurse had read his mind. Differences in values created tension in another relationship when the client had trouble accepting that his nurse was pregnant and yet still continued to work.

Mutual Withdrawal

When the relationship did not progress, there was increasingly limited communication, and the communication remained on a superficial level. Counseling sessions, even when scheduled, would not occur. If sessions did occur, they would be short and frequently set in a public location, such as a hallway. Clients portrayed a relationship of distance, experiencing a wall between themselves and the nurse, and wanting nothing more to do with the nurse. This pattern of mutual withdrawal echoed the concept described decades earlier on an inpatient psychiatric ward by Gwen Tudor (1952).

Nature of the Relationship

The descriptions given about the nurse–client relationship varied considerably between relationships that moved relatively quickly to a working phase compared to those that remained in orientation. When the relationship was in the working phase, clients described closeness, genuine liking, and trust with the nurse. These clients found discussions with their nurses to be safe and easy, and the nurses to be dependable and interested. They reported the nurse's "special attention" and "being there" as important. While they described their nurses as friendly and sociable, they differentiated their relationship with nurses from friendships by noting the relationship as asymmetrical in nature. For example, one client said he did not know what his nurse's house looked like. Another client reported that she would not ask the nurse if she's having an affair but that the nurse could know these things about the client. Other clients stated, "When the client goes home [is discharged] the nurse goes back to her whole life," and "The nurse works for me, I don't work for her."

Several clients discussed the importance of having a good relationship with both their primary and backup nurse. One client commented that having a nurse of each gender was very "powerful," particularly in understanding marital problems. When the relationship remained in the orientation phase for an extended period, a very different description emerged. Clients described "a wall," mutual avoidance, and not talking. One client said she "talks to everybody but nobody listens." These clients described their nurses as if they were not real persons. For example, a client referred to "the nurse" instead of calling him by name. Both clients in orientation beyond six months described not knowing, or caring, if the nurse was on the ward on a particular day.

Discussion

Implications

The results of this study are consistent with Peplau's theory of interpersonal nursing (1991). It is clear from this research that clients place importance on the therapeutic relationship. Peplau (1962, 1965, 1987, 1989d) described this importance as the crux or the heart of nursing. Clients also validated the concept of phases of the nurse–client relationship when they described "moving to a new level." Roles of the nurse identified by the subjects included counseling and liaison/coordinator. A friendship role was not identified. The mutual contributions and interactions of both the nurse and client contributed to progress, or lack of progress, in the therapeutic relationship. In describing the phases of the relationship, we may need to explicitly consider the process as the relationship develops, as well as the process toward mutual withdrawal and impasse when relationships do not work out well.

Clients commented frequently about the need for mutual trust and respect. These needs were met through active listening, consistency, and follow-through. Since availability of the nurse was important, improved scheduling and consistent assignment of nurses should be considered. Some relationships did not progress beyond the orientation phase and became very uncomfortable for clients. Clinical supervision may help resolve impasses. Findings in an earlier study by Forchuk (1995) suggest that if the relationship does not develop within a reasonable amount of time, even with supervision, it would be wise to change the primary nurse. Findings also supported the earlier work by Frank and Gunderson (1990) that if the relationship did not enter the working phase by six months, it was unlikely to do so at all.

Conclusion

The importance that clients placed on the therapeutic relationship reaffirms its importance to nursing practice. Descriptions of the relationship varied greatly, from being "powerful" and "wonderful" in relationships that progressed to the working phase, to being in "limbo" when they did not.

Nurses must attend to what happens between therapeutic sessions, as well as what happens during the planned sessions, to facilitate movement to the working phase. The perceived attitude of the nurse can be viewed as a helping factor or barrier by clients. Behaviors in the nurse such as active listening, trusting, being interested, consistent, and friendly, were valued by participants in this study; however, clients perceived a "superior attitude" and a sense of distance as barriers.

The problem of unavailability is a difficult, multidimensional issue. Shift rotations and client assignments must be planned to support consistent therapeutic relationships. Nurses must make a personal commitment to remaining emotionally available to their clients. Unavailability can develop into a therapeutic impasse and create mutual withdrawal. It is important that nurses recognize these negative patterns and seek clinical supervision or plan a therapeutic client transfer before clients feel "invisible" or "in limbo."

Acknowledgments

Funding Groups: Neimieir Fund, McMaster University; Iota Omicron, Sigma Theta Tau; Lambda Pi, Sigma Theta Tau; and Ontario Hospital Alumnae Association. Consultants to project: Dr. M. M. Leininger and Dr. H. Peplau.

Part III

Care Provider Perspectives

This section details the development and evolution of the therapeutic relationship through the perspective of the care provider. The perspective of care providers is as important to consider as care recipients, since both are partners in the relationship. In my discussions over the years with Dr. Peplau, she frequently said that if the nurse was not assessing himself/herself to the same extent that they were assessing the client, then they are simply not using her theory. For example, it is not enough to note that the client is having difficulty with losses without also reflecting on how one has personally faced losses and to understand how these experiences could promote or interfere with meeting the client's needs.

Chapter 2 in Part I reported on an empirical test of Peplau's theory. Findings demonstrated that information from both partners is needed to fully understand how relationships develop. Both sensitivity and self-reflection are important to forming a strong therapeutic relationship.

In Chapter 5, we find "A Review of Our Understanding of the Care Provider Perspective" by Amy Lewis. This chapter reviews the literature on the care provider role in the development of the therapeutic relationship. It discusses attitudes and approaches that support or hinder these relationships, as well as issues related to transitions in relationships.

Chapter 6 is a reprint of "The Developing Nurse–Client Relationship: Nurses' Perspectives" by Cheryl Forchuk, Jan Westwell, Mary-Lou Martin, Wendy Azzopardi, Donna Kosterewa-Tolman, and Margaret Hux [previously published as Forchuk, C., Westwell, J., Martin, M. L., Bamber-Azzapardi[1], W., Kosterewa-Tolman, D., & Hux, M. (2000). The developing nurse-client relationship: Nurses' perspectives. *Journal of the American Psychiatric Nurses Association*, 6 (1), 3–10. https://doi.org/10.1177%2F107839030000600102]. This chapter parallels Chapter 4 on the client perspective from the qualitative study involving interviews with nurses and clients in the development of therapeutic and non-therapeutic relationships. The focus here is on interviews with nurses. This study confirmed that therapeutic relationships evolve through phases as identified by Peplau and also identified that non-therapeutic relationships evolve though identifiable phases.

Note

1 Previous publication misspelled Azzopardi.

5 A Review of Our Understanding of the Care Provider Perspective

Amy Lewis

Relational transitions happen frequently in healthcare as clients move between inpatient and outpatient settings, among primary, acute, tertiary, and community care contexts, and between different healthcare providers. The role of healthcare providers during these transitions is important to include as providers are responsible for establishing, maintaining, and terminating the therapeutic relationship (College of Nurses of Ontario, 2006). The quality of the therapeutic relationship and the skills that providers bring to the relationship significantly impact client outcomes (Cameron et al., 2018; Cheng et al., 2019; Horvath, 2001). Since providers have an essential function in the therapeutic relationship, this chapter will focus on their role within this dynamic, including the impact of provider attitudes, beliefs, and assumptions, as well as approaches that can support or hinder its development.

The Role of Healthcare Providers in the Therapeutic Relationship

As described in Chapter 1, the therapeutic relationship has three distinct, overlapping phases: the orientation phase, the working phase, and the termination phase (Peplau, 1988a). The role of the provider in each phase of the therapeutic relationship is discussed in more detail below. In relation to each phase, this chapter includes issues and considerations related to the perspectives of providers, as well as evidence-informed activities that are helpful in addressing concerns related to attitudes, beliefs, and assumptions within the therapeutic relationship.

The Orientation Phase

During the orientation phase, the role of the provider is emphasized. It is within this phase that initial trust is established and then tested by the client and where it is important for the provider to demonstrate consistency and clarity regarding their professional role (Forchuk, 1992a). The provider starts by introducing themselves to the client, obtaining a client history, and then getting to know the client before transitioning to the working phase of the relationship (Peplau, 1997). Both the client and the provider enter the orientation phase with preconceptions about one another and expectations for the therapeutic relationship (Peplau, 1997).

The Working Phase

The working phase includes two subphases: identification and exploitation (Peplau, 1988a). During the identification subphase, the client and provider identify problems to work on and develop a plan of care (Registered Nurses' Association of Ontario [RNAO], 2002/2006). Meanwhile, the exploitation subphase involves exploring the thoughts, feelings, and behaviours that the client experiences while implementing the plan of care (RNAO, 2002/2006). Providers take on an active role during this phase by delivering physical care, providing health teaching, conducting interviews and assessments, and counseling the client (Peplau, 1997).

The Termination Phase

In the termination phase, the therapeutic relationship ends. Endings can result from the achievement of goals, transfers in care, relationship transitions, or the death of the client. Healthcare providers have a role in supporting clients to cope with these transitions, such as providing information to combat unfamiliar situations or intervening to alleviate stress (Peplau, 1997).

Attitudes, Beliefs, and Assumptions

It is important to first understand what is meant by attitudes, beliefs, and assumptions. An attitude has cognitive (beliefs), affective (emotive/evaluative), and behavioural (intention) components that are either positive or negative in nature and formed in response to a person, object, or situation (Holden & Smith, 2018). While attitudes are formed *after* a particular experience or interaction, preconceptions are judgments that are made *beforehand*. Beliefs are simply the acceptance of something to be true (Merriam-Webster, n.d.-b). Assumptions are facts or statements that can be taken for granted (Merriam-Webster, n.d.-a). Attitudes, beliefs, and assumptions are critical to address as, under the right conditions, they are influencers of behaviour (see Maio & Haddock, 2010).

Attitudes

Attitudes are formed at an early age through the influences of social learning, repeated exposure to information, and through Pavlovian (classical) and Skinnerian (operant) conditioning (Holden & Smith, 2018). They are also formed upon having immediate experience with an attitude object that is influenced by situational context (Fazio, 1986). Attitudes come from a larger system of values and beliefs that can be traced to religious and moral roots (Miserandino, 2007). Both direct (e.g., new information) and indirect (e.g., persuasion) experiences can reinforce or alter the attitudes that people hold (Holden & Smith, 2018). For instance, attitudes can be influenced by positively or negatively framing events (Van Kleef et al., 2015). An example of this influence involves hearing staff describe clients positively or negatively, which can impact perceptions toward those clients, and ultimately, one's behaviour toward the client. While attitudes can influence behaviour, they are not the sole determinant of behaviour. Social norms, such as perceiving an individual to have power or thinking about the potential consequences of expressing one's attitude through behaviour, also influence actions (Fazio, 1986). It is important to be mindful that clients are quite perceptive to the attitudes and receptiveness of providers, which can impact their own attitudes and experiences in the therapeutic relationship (Easter et al., 2016). In this sense, the attitudes of providers can form a barrier to clients seeking care (Chilale et al., 2017).

Beliefs

Beliefs, as described, are the acceptance of something to be true. Kennedy et al. (2017) compared what providers perceived to be important to clients with what clients reported as their beliefs and values. They also explored whether improving providers' understanding of the client perspective would lead to improvements in communication. Seven providers and 54 clients completed surveys and structured focus groups. The researchers found that providers' beliefs and values differed from those of clients. For instance, clients reported greater meaning than providers in having illness, while providers placed less importance than clients on partnering in care. Clients reported that the most significant factor impacting therapeutic communication was having a shared understanding through bidirectional communication.

Assumptions

Assumptions are cultivated in a number of ways and can influence how providers and clients interact with each other. For example, people who have mental illness are often assumed to be violent and unpredictable (Happell et al., 2019); however, evidence shows that people living with severe mental illness are 11 times more likely to be victims of crime than the general public (Teplin et al., 2006). Such unchallenged assumptions can create harm through fear-based behaviours. Providers may also assume that clients have access to resources. For example, clients who do not have health insurance may not be able to afford prescription medication or community-based therapies. Therefore, it is important that providers ask questions and work collaboratively with clients to ensure goals are realistic and achievable.

Stigma

Stigma consists of both negative attitudes and discriminatory behaviour (Centre for Addiction and Mental Health, n.d.). Specifically, stigma includes "elements of labeling, stereotyping, separation, status loss, and discrimination" that "co-occur in a power situation" (Link & Phelan, 2001, p. 367). The therapeutic relationship between the provider and client, including the family of the client, is one that involves an unequal balance of power (RNAO, 2002/2006). Providers have access to resources, such as knowledge, material provisions, treatments, and other providers, and can even override clients' decision-making if they determine safety is at risk (e.g., involuntarily admitting clients under the *Mental Health Act*; ordering restraints). Meanwhile, clients seek out the provider to access supports and engage in helpful treatment. Providers can mitigate this power differential by using therapeutic communication techniques that include elements of Robert Carkhuff's model, the eight core dimensions of helping (i.e., genuineness, respect, empathy, concreteness, warmth, confrontation, immediacy, and self-disclosure; Stuart, 2009) in the context of shared decision-making. The aim of shared decision-making is to enhance healthcare outcomes by supporting clients' acceptance and engagement in healthcare interventions; however, some tensions exist with using this approach (Slade, 2017).

Providers are trained professionals who are a trusted resource for clients, but unfortunately, they are not immune to holding stigmatizing beliefs. In fact, the attitudes and beliefs held by providers toward people with psychiatric diagnoses do not significantly differ from the views held by the general public (Hansson et al., 2013). Two thirds of people with mental illness avoid seeking treatment primarily because of stigma (Mental Health Commission of Canada [MHCC], 2013). Happell et al. (2019) used a mixed-methods approach to explore the attitudes and perspectives of nursing students toward individuals who have a mental illness. Like Hansson et al. (2013), these researchers found that stigmatizing beliefs were present among the students – even among those who chose a mental health specialization. The sources of stereotypes included fellow nursing staff, family, friends, the media, and ideas developed from their own clinical experiences.

Addressing Attitudes, Beliefs, and Assumptions

While everyone has attitudes, beliefs, and assumptions, there are several ways to challenge potentially harmful ones. Educational institutions can prepare students by engaging them with people who share stories of experience (Happell et al., 2019; Nyblade et al., 2019). When 'Experts by Experience' were involved in developing and delivering modules about mental illness to nursing students, the students felt challenged to reflect on their attitudes and beliefs and to think more critically about delivering mental healthcare (Happell et al., 2019). *De-Stigmatizing Practices and Mental Illness* is a free online course available from www.mdcme.ca that includes both educational and reflective activities.

Both skills training and programs that include contact with Experts by Experience support providers to develop positive attitudes and behaviours toward people who have mental illness (MHCC, 2013). Journaling is a more private and individualized approach. The Alberta Health Services (n.d.) has adapted questions from different trauma-informed toolkits that can facilitate reflective activity. An important step of any reflective practice is identifying what needs to change and taking action to achieve that change.

Recovery-Oriented Approaches

The recovery-oriented perspective began surfacing in the 1980s and 1990s by people with personal experience who wanted a system that instilled hope, treated people with respect and dignity, and supported personal well-being (MHCC, 2015). A recovery-oriented approach does not mean curing the person. Instead, it involves recognizing that each person is the expert of their own life, with clients working in partnership with the provider to make choices in their journey that builds on their strengths and abilities (Australian Government Department of Health, 2010).

Providers can easily take a 'futility perspective' when they rarely see clients recover in ways that they anticipate. Consider this quote from a psychiatric nurse:

> Another point is that I saw its futility. I mean the same repeated hospitalizations; they go and come back; I personally do not see the result of my job. I can't see that at least one patient has recovered, got home, and now he/she leads his/her own life; very rarely. Well, I say what difference does it make to establish a relationship with these patients or not? (P. No. 5).
>
> (Pazargadi et al., 2015, p. 554)

Notice how the nurse expected that clients were able to go home and lead their own lives? The nurse also questioned whether it was worthwhile to develop a therapeutic relationship. What remains unknown is the context of care, such as the approaches that the nurses used and the organizational resources to support this work.

Provider attitudes and beliefs and the context of care can act as facilitators or barriers to developing the therapeutic relationship. The provision of healthcare has traditionally been paternalistic, where clients were expected to follow professional medical advice; however, people have unique needs and capabilities that must be incorporated in the plan of care, which further reinforces a partnership approach. Some providers still emphasize the illness-based model and strive to have clients accept their symptoms and limitations (Easter et al., 2016). Recovery-oriented approaches situate the beliefs of the provider to be in line with the strengths of the person receiving care, rather than with provider expectations.

Multiple guidelines and conceptual models of recovery-oriented approaches exist. In Canada, recovery-oriented practice has six key dimensions (MHCC, 2015): creating a culture and language of hope; recovery is personal; recovery occurs in the context of one's life; responding to the diverse needs of everyone living in Canada; working with First Nations, Inuit, and Metis; and recovery is about transforming services and systems. A framework that applies more broadly is conceptualized under the acronym CHIME, which stands for connectedness, hope and optimism, identity, meaning and purpose, and empowerment (Leamy et al., 2011).

Facilitators and Barriers to the Therapeutic Relationship: Healthcare Provider Roles

Multiple factors contribute to the ability of the provider to deliver care and work in partnership with clients. Among clients with mental illness, factors that facilitate the therapeutic relationship include client-focused goal setting, the time and availability of treatment providers, using a caring approach, and establishing trust and honesty in the relationship (Easter et al., 2016). Providers can support the interpersonal nature of the therapeutic relationship by using therapeutic listening, responding to clients' emotions and unmet needs, and emphasizing client-centredness (Kornhaber et al., 2016).

Providers also experience numerous barriers to forming the therapeutic relationship and in providing mental healthcare. Lack of time is still a fundamental concern, with providers in different settings experiencing varying types of time constraints. For providers in primary care, the time available to meet with each client is minimal, so the provision of emotional support may be delegated to other staff or not provided at all (Poghosyan et al., 2019). Meanwhile, providers who work in mental health settings may feel pressured to balance collecting enough information with ensuring the client has enough time to express themselves (Nakash et al., 2018).

Within psychiatric wards, nurses identified three categories of barriers to the therapeutic relationship: nurse-related barriers, patient-related barriers, and organizational barriers (Pazargadi et al., 2015). Nurse-related barriers included negative personal characteristics of the nurse (e.g., aggressive characteristics), work exhaustion (e.g., tiredness and job dissatisfaction), inadequate skills (e.g., inexperience with psychosis, inadequate communication skills), pattern-taking (i.e., following the trends of other nurses' practice), and negative attitude of nurses (e.g., fear that interacting with people who have mental illness could personally affect the nurse). Patient-related barriers involved characteristics of clients that interfered with therapeutic communication, such as lack of knowledge and inability to communicate with others.

Organizational barriers were the most significant issue and included workplace conditions, such as manpower shortage, a large number of patients, and work overload, all of which reduced the availability of nurses to interact with clients. Within the relationship dynamic, the priorities of providers and clients can differ significantly (e.g., clients prioritized finding housing, while providers prioritized the treatment of denial; Easter et al., 2016). In some cases, this difference was so powerful that it led to clients disengaging with services. Supportive, open communication between the provider and client is a necessary facilitator to identifying problems and working to resolve them (Forchuk & Reynolds, 2001).

Conclusion

In reviewing the literature for this chapter, it was found that more research is needed from the perspective of healthcare providers regarding their attitudes, beliefs, and assumptions. Attitudes, beliefs, and assumptions play a critical role in the therapeutic relationship through their potential influence over clinical decision-making and actions. A number of programs and activities exist to help students and providers identify and address potentially harmful attitudes, beliefs, and assumptions, such as hearing stories from people with personal experience, involving Experts by Experience in educational program design and delivery, and incorporating reflective practice. Recovery-oriented approaches also provide frameworks to keep provider beliefs in line with the strengths of the client. Providers and clients may place different emphasis on what they perceive to be important, so providers should take the lead to explore and incorporate what clients consider to be most valuable in terms of communication, co-creating the plan of care, and implementing the plan of care.

6   The Developing Nurse–Client Relationship

Nurses' Perspectives

Cheryl Forchuk, Jan Westwell, Mary-Lou Martin,
Wendy Azzopardi, Donna Kosterewa-Tolman, and
Margaret Hux

Nursing theorist Hildegard Peplau described the nurse–client relationship as evolving through interlocking, overlapping phases (1952/1991). The first phase of the relationship, the orientation phase, occurs when the nurse and client first meet as strangers and develop mutual trust. This trust develops as the client tests the parameters of the relationship and the nurse consistently and appropriately responds to this testing. The relationship moves into the working phase when the client participates in the identification of problems and subproblems (Peplau, 1952/1991). The duration of the orientation phase varies considerably, lasting from minutes to months (Forchuk, 1993). However, dyads in which the client has a chronic mental illness frequently have orientation phases of six months or longer (Forchuk, 1992a).

Silva (1986) has discussed the infrequent testing of nursing theories. Although Peplau's theory has been reported as the most common nursing theory used in psychiatric-mental health practice by both Canadian (Martin & Kirkpatrick, 1987, 1989) and American (Hirschmann, 1989) surveys, Peplau's theoretical framework, like other nursing theories, has seldom been tested.

Purpose and Questions

The purpose was to describe the evolving nurse–client relationship from the nurses' perspective and to then compare the described patterns with those in Peplau's theory. To address this purpose, the research questions from the nurses' perspectives included the following:

1. What is the nature of the relationship?
2. How are therapeutic relationships progressing?
3. What seems to be helping the development of a therapeutic relationship?
4. What seems to be hampering the development of a therapeutic relationship?

Methods

This descriptive qualitative study used an interpersonal focus and Leininger's (1985) method of qualitative analysis. The analysis included identifying and listing descriptors of observations, combining descriptors into patterns, synthesizing patterns into larger holistic themes, and testing themes by reviewing raw data (Leininger, 1985).

The setting was a tertiary care psychiatric hospital in southern Ontario, Canada. Ethical approval was received from the hospital research committee. Nurses and clients in newly formed dyads participated in separate audiotaped interviews throughout the orientation phase.

Nurse–client interactions were also observed and videotaped. This report focuses on nurses' perceptions of the evolving nurse–client relationships as shared in the audiotaped interviews.

Results

Description of Participants

Ten nurse–client dyads participated in the study. The clients, six men and four women, were receiving inpatient care from a tertiary care psychiatric facility. Clients were diagnosed with either schizophrenia (n=7) or a mood disorder (n=3). The nurses were all registered and each possessed more than ten years of psychiatric nursing experience. Two of the nurses were male and both formed dyads with male clients. The four female clients and four male clients had female nurses.

Nature and Development of Relationships

Some relationships progressed well, whereas others encountered difficulties. Seven dyads were able to establish a working relationship during the admission. The time required for this varied between 2.5 weeks to six months. Two dyads did not reach a working relationship, although they continued to attempt this for almost one year before switching the nurse assignment. One client was discharged after six months, and a working relationship was never formed with the nurse. Relationships that were described as working well involved regular, frequent, and private interactions, which led to feelings of trust and the ability to share problems. Relationships were described as part of the team approach. After they established trust and shared problems, a gradual weaning process that tied in with the discharge process took place. Sometimes telephone contact was maintained after formal discharge. Words used to describe these working relationships were "comfortable," "smooth," "cooperative," and "honest." One nurse described the relationship as "very relaxed from the beginning. I think, in some way, I am with him." Another stated, "I'm the one person who's constant and he feels comfortable talking with…." Another nurse said, "I really enjoy this relationship. I really enjoy working with [client]." When relationships were not working well, nurses described clients as "difficult," "frustrating," "superficial," and "not co-operative." Nurses felt a lack of communication and tended to blame the client for difficulties in the relationship. Examples of comments include, "He sees me as the type of person he comes to if he needs cigarettes," and "I think that he is too lazy to want to work through problems and would be happy just to, kind of, not use me in a good therapeutic way if he doesn't have to."

The pattern of relationships often started the same, but numerous, changing strategies were introduced when relationships did not progress. It seemed that the nurse was grappling with what to do next. These strategies include being more or less directive, varying the duration of the interaction, or varying the therapeutic stance. When relationships did not progress, nurses and clients became increasingly frustrated. Comments illustrating this frustration include, "No matter how I deal with those answers I'm still getting the same questions over and over again…that sort of frustration comes," and "I don't think it makes me feel angry. I think it just makes me feel like that, um, like I'm not mad at him or I'm not angry with him. I just feel that I could do so many other things and not have to worry about him."

As the level of frustration increased, the members of the dyad began to avoid each other. Tudor (1952) described this process as "mutual withdrawal." Interactions became less formal, less private, and shorter. The classic in-hall, brief encounter was typical. Nurses' comments include:

Well, I usually see [client] maybe 5 times a day. But it's only for a couple of minutes.

Unchangeable. The same. I give him a couple of minutes to get warmed up, then I just cut it short.

I don't really do interviews anymore…it's just short, frequent contacts.

The pattern was to blame the client for the failure of the relationship, as the following comments illustrate:

The reason for the difficulty to follow through is the motivation…I think he's also a very isolating person.

I don't think it's he and I who are having this problem. I think he would be like this with any of my coworkers, judging from some of the things I hear in the report and at change of shift time.

The nurse did not consider the difficult situation as a typical example of his or her relationship with clients. In the study, three cases exemplified the difficult non-progressing relationship. In two of these cases, the difficulties were resolved when the client began to work with a different nurse.

Helping Factors

From the nurses' perspectives, certain behaviors were beneficial to the progression of the nurse–client relationship. These were grouped as nurse factors: consistency, pacing, listening; interactional factors: initial impression, comfort and control; and client factors.

Consistency

Consistency was a recurring theme that was reflected in many ways. Having a nurse assigned consistently to the same client helped make the client more comfortable. When the client's primary nurse was not available, the presence of a backup or planned associate nurse became important. It was necessary for this associate nurse to have good rapport with the client and with the primary nurse. A regular routine for activities of daily living and interactions was needed, and orientation to the routine was seen as important. Interactions were facilitated by being frequent and regular in duration, format, and location. As one nurse said, "I think the contact with me being the primary nurse and the consistency of seeing [client] everyday, the associate nurse, and the consistent times set up for our interaction daily helped quite a bit."

Nurses declared that even clients in psychotic states were well aware of their appointments, able to identify their nurse, and able to recognize their existing relationships. One nurse said, "Even in his psychotic state he identified me as his nurse, as opposed to the countless other people he could be talking to." Nurses spoke of being honest and consistent in what they were saying to the client; some nurses linked honesty with openness. These characteristics were also linked to clients' degree of receptiveness to help and their efforts. One nurse stated, "I admitted him and told him right then that I'm the admitting nurse and I'll be his nurse from now until he's discharged." A second nurse stated she was one of the first people seen when the client was admitted and, therefore, seemed to be the client's primary contact. Another nurse spoke of being "available for all meetings [the client] attended." This enabled the nurse to make appropriate referrals when required. The nurse saw the way one responded to initial requests as very important in developing the relationship.

Pacing

A slow approach reduced pressure and was seen to be an enabling force for the development of the relationship. Nurses felt the pace should be set by the client and should be adjusted to the client's mood. It may be necessary for the nurse to "stand back and realize that things will take a long time and one needs to take one day at a time." In other instances, it may be essential to leave clients until they have "settled down and are ready to talk."

Listening

The third theme identified was the importance of listening. Inherent in this theme is the idea of letting the client talk. One nurse stated that the interactions were not taking place to share information but to let the client talk, as this was the client's need. The nurse was to be a sounding board. Consequently, the client was doing most of the talking; the nurse's role was "not to confront." When it was necessary to mention hallucinations, the nurse thought it was appropriate to comment on the behaviors observed by saying something such as, "I notice you talking to yourself."

Initial Impression

Preconceptions and positive initial attitudes were seen as significant considerations. One nurse spoke of knowing the client from a previous admission; "we just fit in," said the nurse. The nurse was also aware of the client's patterns. Some nurses described clients as being "interesting" or "challenging." These ideas stemmed from the length of time the clients had been in hospital and the presentation of their symptoms. Nurses spoke of expecting progress and positive outcomes. An early comment from one nurse was, "We're getting along really well... She's trying really hard."

Comfort and Control

Other nurses suggested promoting client comfort and balancing control, which would demonstrate caring behaviors. Acknowledging the client's familiarity with the therapeutic process, as in the case where the client knew the facility and had been a therapist herself, was also seen as helpful. Absence of confrontation was seen as important at this stage of the relationship. A familiar face was seen as helpful. One nurse said, "When he was here before, he saw my face around; I was familiar, I think that helped." Control was considered to be based on balancing: "it should not be too strict and not too lenient, I keep a firm hold."

Client Factors

Nurses found it useful when clients actively participated in the therapeutic process and when clients could trust the nurse. One nurse stated, "She comes to me and understands our relationship now...that I am her primary nurse and [she] seeks out, you know, her needs." Another nurse said, "I think she trusts me. Like when she needs something or wants to talk about something, she knows I'm available for her...whenever I'm on."

Hampering Factors

Nurses deduced that hampering factors in the development of positive relationships centered on inconsistency and unavailability, nurses' feelings and lack of self-awareness, patient factors and trust, confrontation of delusions, and unrealistic expectations. These factors interacted to create a negative environment and avoidance on the part of both the nurse and the client.

Inconsistency and Unavailability

Inconsistency and unavailability related to various areas including interactions, nursing goals, and different realities. Almost all nurses complained about the time constraints, scheduling, and organizational issues that interfered with their ability to meet with clients. Nurses complained about time constraints around availability for meetings, missed appointments, and lack of contact with clients.

In the relationships that did not progress to a therapeutic level, this lack of availability and inconsistency went beyond the level of organizational issues and were more specific to the dyad. The lack of contact included infrequent meetings, meeting in the hallway, and the clients' reluctance or refusal to sit and talk with nurses. One nurse stated, "There is no point in dragging him to a special place when he's not going to talk anyway."

Nurses also addressed missed appointments stating, "he doesn't keep the appointments... then it seems kind of pointless." Other nurses addressed the deliberate missing of appointments by saying, "I will set up the appointment time to meet him, he'll either fall asleep or he'll go out for a walk and not bother coming back." This lack of availability is a major feature of the "mutual avoidance" phase of relationships that did not progress in a therapeutic manner.

Nurses' Feelings and Awareness

Another theme that emerged from the nurses' interviews was lack of self-awareness and the nurses' own feelings. The nurses talked about preconceived ideas and about feelings of discomfort, dislike of clients, fear, and avoidance. They also spoke of the effects of inappropriate pacing and lack of progress. One nurse talked about rushing in and confusing the client. The nurse withdrew and stayed away longer from the client as a result of the painful nature of the interaction. When talking about feeling uncomfortable in the presence of the client, one nurse had difficulties in handling personal questions from a client: "It's more of a gut feeling, you know, because he has this kind of look about him when he asks these [personal] questions as opposed to when we're talking [in a] normal type of conversation." This nurse later said,

> I've never told him these questions make me uncomfortable. I have told him that they are inappropriate in the context of what we are discussing and in our work relationship that we have....I don't think I really explore in depth my feelings about it or...I've never really analyzed why I think he's asking me these questions.

The nurse did not see herself as helping and stated that she needed to "re-orient" her thinking.

A nurse mentioned, "I just can't feel sympathetic toward this guy, and I think I never will." One nurse also expressed fear of the client. The nurse stated, "I was becoming really afraid of him because he was becoming very overt...just telling me freely that he wanted to kiss me and touch me...." The same nurse felt apprehensive and on guard around the client and did not feel comfortable being alone with the client. Lack of progress in the relationship and avoidance were other factors about which the nurses expressed concern. In some circumstances, nurses felt that during the interactions that happened, they, the nurse and client, were "just going through the motions." "This is a kind of stagnation; it really brings me down," explained one nurse. Nurses also described the interactions as "going in circles." This led nurses to feel useless, which gave way to avoidance. The nurse spoke of not wanting to have anything to do with the client and also about ways to avoid the client in the hallway.

Patient Factors and Trust

Another area of concern that nurses addressed was labeled patient factors. These were issues surrounding trust or confidentiality, patient responsibility, patient paranoia and delusions, and patient anxiety and anger. Nurses reported that some clients were guarded in their discussions when the subject matter revolved around their well-being because they were concerned that the conversations might be used against them. For example, a client who was on probation for drug trafficking was reluctant to discuss his drug-use history because he believed that by acknowledging current drug use, it would be held against him.

> He doesn't talk to me about the problems he had when he came to hospital. He says, "okay," "fine," "you know it"...[we] never really get into the problem.

Nurses also spoke of the client "trying to gloss over things" and of trying "to deny things." Client anger also hampered the development of the relationship. For example, clients might group all the staff together; consequently, when anger existed toward one staff member, it was displaced against all staff. Nurses also described clients who wanted their needs met immediately. When clients were delusional, relationship damage occurred if the nurse tried confrontation to establish reality, particularly if this approach preceded the establishment of trust.

Another issue related to delusions occurred when the nurse was incorporated into the delusional system. One nurse said, "[according to the client] I was a lawyer and I was responsible for taking his kids away. That's come up three times and he's quite angry about that."

Expectations

One final issue that presented problems to nurses was the idea of expectations. Nurses believed that difficult relationships were not typical for them; therefore, they did not expect their occurrence. The nurses believed most clients should be able to sit down and discuss their problems. Nurses believed their goals differed from the clients' goals. In one instance the nurse stated, "We're not really talking about the things I think are important."

Implications

Consistent, regular, and private interactions with clients were seen as essential to the development of therapeutic relationships. Staffing patterns and client assignments can facilitate or hamper this consistency. Nurses in this study stressed the importance of listening, pacing, and consistency.

The helping factors and description of the therapeutic relationships are consistent with Peplau's theory. However, not all dyads followed Peplau's classic route of orientation phase, working phase (identification and exploitation), and, finally, resolution. It appears the dyads that experienced difficulties started the relationship in the orientation phase, but instead of moving to the working phase, they moved to a mutually frustrating phase in which different approaches were attempted and abandoned. In an effort to define this alternate phase, we have labeled it the "grappling and struggling" phase. From this previous phase, relationships moved to the mutual withdrawal phase. Figure 6.1 illustrates the classic phases of the development of the therapeutic relationship that were observed in seven dyads in this study, as well as the

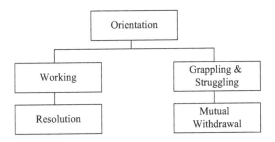

Figure 6.1 Phases of Therapeutic and Non-Therapeutic Relationships. Forchuk, C., Westwell, J., Martin, M.-L., Bamber-Azzapardi, W., Kosterewa-Tolman, D., & Hux, M. (2000). The developing nurse-client relationship: Nurses' perspectives. *Journal of the American Psychiatric Nurses Association*, *6*(1), 3–10. Copyright© (SAGE Publications). https://doi.org/10.1177%2F1078 39030000600102.

alternate route taken by three dyads. The hampering factors can be understood in context of this route to non-therapeutic relationships.

Conclusion

The nature of the relationship as described by Peplau was supported for those relationships that progressed in a mutually satisfying manner. Nevertheless, some relationships appeared to take a more negative alternate path. In this study, phases of both therapeutic and non-therapeutic relationships were observed and analyzed.

Acknowledgments

We thank the consultants to this project: Dr. M. M. Leininger, Dr. H. Peplau.

Part IV

Exploration of Key Concepts

In Part IV, we will explore some key concepts related to therapeutic relationships. Both compassion and empathy can be seen as foundational to relationships.

In Chapter 7, entitled "Compassion as Collaboration" by Kathleen Ledoux, compassion is explored. Compassion, at its most fundamental level, is an expression of both our ability and desire to care. Compassion catalyzes us to understand and, thus, know the other. This chapter focuses on research that demonstrates how compassion enables a provider to be sensitive to and connect with the care recipient. That connection enables collaboration between the receiver and provider. This chapter also discusses the research regarding the barriers and facilitators to the development of compassion among providers.

Chapter 8 is entitled "Empathy: The Core of the Nurse–Client Relationship" and is authored by William Reynolds. Empathy has been considered a foundational concept to establishing relationships. This chapter will describe empathy and differentiate it from similar concepts, such as sympathy and caring. The role of empathy, as well as its measure, is also described.

The next two concepts explored are concepts that could support or undermine the therapeutic relationship. These chapters explore new emerging technologies and ethical issues related to relationships.

Kamini Kalia and Amy Lewis have authored Chapter 9 entitled "New Technologies." New technologies are emerging in health, including phone-based apps, online tools, and virtual care visits. How do these emerging technologies impact relationships? Guidelines for the use of technology that support relationships are included.

Chapter 10 is entitled "Ethics and Boundaries in Therapeutic Relationships" and is authored by Brad A. MacNeil, Cheryl Forchuk, and Abraham Rudnick. Ethical principles are discussed in the context of therapeutic relationships. In particular, boundaries to the therapeutic relationship are explored and guidelines to assist in maintaining appropriate boundaries are outlined. This chapter also includes considerations during transitions in relationships.

7 Compassion as Collaboration

Kathleen Ledoux

This chapter will discuss two key nursing concepts: the therapeutic relationship and compassion. Compassion and the therapeutic relationship appear to be understood, although crucial together, as two stand-alone concepts. The link between compassion, trust, and the formation of the therapeutic relationship will be explored. In addition, evidence will be provided that we each have the capacity to be compassionate and that compassion can be learned and measured.

Compassion

Compassion is regarded as a core component of healthcare (Shea & Lionis, 2017). Frequently, providers, policy makers, professional groups, and healthcare organizations will speak to their aim to provide compassionate care (e.g., the UK's National Health Service [NHS Commissioning Board, 2012], the American Medical Association [AMA Principles of Medical Ethics, 2019], and the International Council of Nurses [2012]). Likewise, patients and their significant others consistently rank compassionate care, along with competent care, to be of the highest importance (Sinclair et al., 2016). There is evidence that compassionate care can enhance recovery, improve management of chronic illnesses, reduce stress and anxiety, and increase pain tolerance (Mannion, 2014; Shea & Lionis, 2017).

Compassion has been examined since at least the time of Aristotle (Cassell, 2002). Despite familiarity with and much use of the term "compassion," there can be a lack of consensus as to what compassion is in its attributes, actions, and effects (Gilbert, 2017; Mannion, 2014). One definition, which has arisen both from the research and from Buddhist philosophy, is that compassion is a sensitivity to suffering with a wish to act to relieve the suffering (Neff, 2003; Tendhar, 2019).

In a review of 20 years of research on compassion, Goetz and colleagues (2010) found compassion to be a distinct "affective state" (p. 354) differing from empathy, sympathy, or pity. Empathy is a mirroring and understanding of another's situation, enabling one to feel similar to or the same as the other person but without a motivational component to act. Sympathy is a feeling of concern but without mirroring (understanding) the other's state. Pity is considered to be closely related to sympathy. It is a feeling of concern, but most typically felt when one feels more powerful than the other with a reluctance to become involved (Keltner & Goetz, 2007). The review revealed that individuals with compassion have a unique assessment process attuned to suffering, an other-orientation with a desire to approach, a willingness to act, and specific methods of caring (e.g., posture, speaking, touch). This desire to approach and to act is compassion's defining characteristic (Chierchia & Singer, 2017). Empathy, sympathy, or pity alone do not motivate one to act (Goetz et al., 2010).

Compassion has three elements: kindness, mindfulness, and common or shared humanity (Gilbert, 2005; Neff, 2003). Kindness is defined as acting with warmth and understanding. Mindfulness is being in a state of equanimity where one is neither over-identified with nor disengaged from the other. It is noticing without avoidance or aversion; paying attention to the experience in the moment. Common humanity is knowing that suffering is a universal human experience. It is understanding that suffering does not discriminate and is a common denominator for all people.

The Psychological and Evolutionary Processes of Compassion

Knowing the definition of and variables that compose compassion does not yet describe what its mechanism of action is. Jazaieri et al. (2013) describe a psychological process (Table 7.1) that takes place as compassion unfolds. These steps do not always progress seamlessly. Perhaps, for example, there is no awareness that suffering is occurring or there is an appraisal that you do not have the resources to respond. In fact, there may be no response, as we tend to express compassion more readily for members of our own group than for strangers (Singer & Klimecki, 2014). Indeed, in the face of suffering, some experience satisfaction, or *schadenfreude*, that the other is suffering (Portman, 2014). An important step is the last: the experience of satisfaction. It has been shown that this feeling helps to condition the compassionate response and encourages future compassionate responses (McGonigal, 2017).

From an evolutionary perspective, it is hypothesized that humans are born to be compassionate (Lown, 2015; Weng et al., 2013). Although defensive behaviours are generally accepted as an evolutionary standard for a species' survival, prosocial behaviours can equally be viewed as having an evolutionary benefit. Compassion may have evolved as a means of survival (Goetz et al., 2010; Sober & Wilson, 1999). It is hypothesized that prosocial behaviours, including compassion, enabled early humans to live safely together and successfully raise their vulnerable offspring (Carter et al., 2017). These caring behaviours have beneficial psychological, social, and health effects that assist in survivability.

Therapeutic Relationship

To understand the dynamic between compassion and the therapeutic relationship, we must now define what the therapeutic relationship is, and like compassion, its components and processes. Peplau (1962) said that the therapeutic relationship is the crux of nursing. Others agree (Glembocki & Fitzpatrick, 2013; Manthey, 2015; McQueen, 2000; O'Brien, 2001). As stated by the Registered Nurses' Association of Ontario (2002/2006), the therapeutic relationship is a "purposeful, goal-oriented relationship that is directed at advancing the best interest and outcome of the patient" (p. 13). It is in the nature of the therapeutic relationship to enable the nurse to provide individualized care (McQueen, 2000). The nurse–patient therapeutic relationship

Table 7.1 Compassion's Process

Steps in the Compassionate Response Process
An awareness/recognition of suffering
A feeling of concern for and a connection to the one who is suffering
A desire to relieve the suffering
A belief that you can make a difference
A willingness to respond/take action
A warm glow/sense of satisfaction

then is a deliberative, collaborative, decision-making partnership that is formed to advance the patient's health, taking into account both the patient's and the nurse's healthcare goals for the patient.

Phases of the Therapeutic Relationship

Peplau's (1962) theory of the therapeutic relationship proposes that there are three phases in establishing a therapeutic relationship: the initial or orientation phase, the working phase, and the resolution phase. The initial phase occurs when the patient and the nurse "come to know each other as persons and the client begins to trust the nurse" (Forchuk, 1993, p. 9). The second or working phase of the relationship is the time when the majority of the work of nursing occurs. Once trust has been established, both the nurse and the patient make full use of the relationship to work on identified goals. Ballatt and Campling (2011) concur that trust generates the therapeutic relationship. The final phase occurs when the problem(s) is resolved. Closure of the relationship occurs at this time.

As the therapeutic relationship is the crux of nursing, then from the above it follows that trust is the crux of the therapeutic relationship – before there can be a therapeutic relationship, there must be trust. Shea and Lionis (2017) concur. Trust leads to nurse–patient collaboration and thus to a "more accurate understanding and diagnosis" (Shea & Lionis, 2017, p. 3). Knowing that trust is crucial to the therapeutic relationship, how does trust arise?

Trustworthiness

To be judged trustworthy in a clinical context, one must have certain qualities. Surprisingly, what makes a person trustworthy is not well understood (Dinc, & Gastmans, 2012; Eriksson & Nilsson, 2008; Thielman & Hilbig, 2015). Research has focused more on why people trust than on what counts as being trustworthy. Those studies that have been done to explore trustworthiness have shown that in order to be considered trustworthy, the clinician must demonstrate not only clinical competence, but also respect, engagement, a willingness to listen, and a non-judgmental disposition (Eriksson & Nilsson, 2008). Murray and McCrone (2015) state the same; one must demonstrate an ability to listen and a desire to understand. Eriksson and Nilsson (2008) add that the quality of calmness encourages trust. On the other hand, depersonalizing and being distant inhibit the formation of trust (Dinc & Gastmans, 2013). Hutchison et al. (2016) in a study examining surrogate decision-makers' judgement of clinicians' trustworthiness, found that clinicians who were benevolent or kind, who were invested, who sought to find common qualities, and presented themselves as "human" were perceived to be trustworthy. Thielman and Hilbig (2015) in three non-clinical studies of the determinants of trustworthiness found that kindness is a quality of trustworthiness.

Compassion, Trustworthiness, and the Therapeutic Relationship

The nature of the nurse–patient therapeutic relationship is described in similar ways as a trusting relationship. Carl Rogers, (McQueen, 2000) considered a founder of person-centered psychotherapy, identified three fundamental qualities in a therapeutic relationship: empathic understanding, unconditional positive regard (acceptance of others as individuals entitled to respect), and genuineness (authenticity) (Scanlon, 2006). To be therapeutic, these qualities were necessarily coupled with the clinician's competence and desire to help (McQueen, 2000). The nursing literature on the nurse–patient therapeutic relationship is in agreement. The nurse in the nurse–patient therapeutic relationship is described as having the qualities of kindness, authenticity, respectfulness, acceptance, being without prejudice, providing individualized care, being understanding, listening, being accessible and available, and showing a commitment to help (Dziopa & Ahern, 2009; Moreno-Poyato et al., 2018; Scanlon, 2006). As seen above, these qualities are the same as the qualities that inspire trust.

From the above descriptions of compassion, trustworthiness, and the therapeutic relationship, it can be seen that the attributes of each concept map on to each other (Table 7.2).

It can be argued that compassion is a catalyst that enables the therapeutic relationship to form, as the attributes of a compassionate person are the same as a trustworthy person. It is trustworthiness that establishes the therapeutic relationship. This seems so clear when the characteristics of one (compassion) are compared to the qualities of the other (trustworthiness). Compassion is not some separate valued quality or attitude, but necessary for the therapeutic relationship to occur.

Barriers to Compassion

Understanding that while compassion is a facilitator of the therapeutic relationship, it is not always the case that compassion is present (Shea et al., 2014). Valdesolo and DeSteno (2011) found that compassion is not felt by all people at all times. As shown earlier (Table 7.1), the expression of compassion has certain requirements, which if unfulfilled, will impede its expression. The desire to relieve suffering may be additionally confounded by what Gilbert and Mascaro (2017) describe as fears, blocks, and resistance (Table 7.3).

Further, Ledoux and colleagues (2018) found that insufficient organizational support, lack of resources (both time and staff), uncertain nurse decisional authority, lack of information, poor interprofessional collaboration, poor self-efficacy, and a poor fit with the organization's goals

Table 7.2 Comparison of Compassion, Trustworthiness, and Therapeutic Relationship Attributes

	Compassion	Trustworthiness	Therapeutic Relationship
Kindness			
	Considerate	Kindness	Understanding
	Interested	Benevolence	Accepting
	Understanding	Desire to understand	Kind
	Non-critical (accepting)	Invested	
	Not harsh (gentle)		
Mindfulness			
	Choosing to pay attention	Engagement	Listening
	A state of equanimity	Willingness to listen	Accessible
	Paying attention without avoidance/ aversion	Calmness	Available
			Authentic
Common Humanity			
	Understands all humans share common attributes	Respect	Respect
	Views other as an individual; non-stereotyping/dehumanizing/ stigmatizing	Non-judgemental	Individualized care
		Common qualities/ Humanness	Absence of prejudice

Table 7.3 Fears, Blocks, and Resistance to Compassion

Fears

- People will take advantage of me
- People will think I'm weak
- Needy people will be drawn to me and will drain my emotional resources

Blocks

- Do not have the resources
- Do not have the power
- Dehumanize the other

Resistance

- Competing motivations
- Believe discipline and punishment are more helpful than compassion

all have a negative effect on the ability to practice compassionately. Similarly, Brown et al. (2014) and Gilbert and Mascaro (2017) identified that lack of leadership, interpersonal conflicts, work stress, routinized care, and role confusion hinder compassionate care. The requirement to meet external performance targets and an overemphasis on efficiency can also hamper compassionate care (Mannion, 2014). If all of these things inhibit compassion, then they all inhibit the therapeutic relationship. Fortunately, each of these barriers might be overcome or at least mitigated by attending to their opposite.

Compassion: Measurable and Learnable

While mitigating for the above barriers may be challenging or perhaps in some instances, not possible, it *is* possible to attend to the self to develop and strengthen one's innate compassionate response, which increases the likelihood of establishing the therapeutic relationship – even in the face of such challenges. Compassion can be learned and measured (Lown et al., 2015). Jazaieri et al. (2013), in a randomized control trial, found that following a nine-week compassion cultivation course, participants in the intervention group had significant increases in all three domains of compassion (compassion for others, self-compassion, and receiving compassion) compared to the control group. Brito-Pons and colleagues (2018) in a randomized controlled trial found the same outcomes, but within a different population. Weng et al., (2013) similarly found that after a two-week compassion training program that compassion was cultivated. Finally, a systematic review and meta-analysis of randomized controlled studies of the effect of meditation training on empathy, compassion, and pro-social behaviours also showed improvements in compassionate behaviours (Luberto et al., 2018).

Conclusion

Both compassion and the therapeutic relationship are considered essential in care. From the preceding, we have discovered how the attributes of compassion are similar to the attributes of trustworthiness. As trust is the crux of the therapeutic relationship, the compassionate clinician would then be more capable of developing a therapeutic relationship. Ledoux et al. (2018) found that the motivation and ability to be compassionate is contingent on both environmental and personal influences. However, compassion can be learned and enhanced to help overcome challenges to the formation of the therapeutic relationship.

It is with this new-found understanding that this chapter ends, reflecting that we consider education in compassion as central in assisting nurses to be able to develop the therapeutic relationship.

8 Empathy

The Core of the Nurse–Client Relationship

William Reynolds

Empathy is often seen as crucial to all forms of helping relationships (Reynolds, 2009). While empathy is commonly described as an ability to communicate an understanding of another's world, there is confusion about whether empathy is a personality dimension, an experienced emotion, or an observable skill. This chapter will review the multidimensional nature of empathy. Additionally, it will discuss the role of empathy in clinical nursing and how it is measured.

The Relevance of Empathy to the Purpose of the Nurse–Client Relationship

Truax (1970) emphasized that without empathy, there is no basis for appreciating the client perspective and responding in ways that result in favourable health outcomes. This view has been repeated by others who have pointed to the voluminous amount of the research and theoretical findings supporting that empathy is the critical ingredient of helping relationships (e.g., Altwalbeh et al., 2018; Reynolds, 2000; Rogers, 1975; Yu & Kirk, 2009).

It is useful to review the intended outcomes of the nurse-client relationship. For example, Kalkman (1967) referred to the nurse–client relationship as relationship therapy "during which the patient can feel accepted as a person of worth, feels free to express him/herself, and is enabled to learn more satisfactory and productive patterns of living" (p. 266). Congruent with that view, Forchuk and Reynolds (2001) identified three aims of the nurse–client relationship, which are:

- Initiating supportive interpersonal communication in order to understand the needs of the other person.
- Empowering the other person to learn or cope more effectively with their environment.
- Reducing or resolving the problems of another person.

Arguably, these outcomes are relevant to all nurse–client relationships, but they are critical in psychiatric nursing contexts. Peplau (1988b) proposed that the phenomena observed by psychiatric nurses during their relationships with clients should be the focus for nursing interventions. Peplau suggested that the focus includes a considerable array of human response patterns including anxiety, disorientation, hallucinations, delusional ideation, negative self-concept, loneliness, and passive-aggressiveness. Peplau also stated that psychiatric nurses have unparalleled opportunity to make themselves experts in a humanistic alternative approach to such problems. Humanistic refers to the value of human beings individually and a tendency to believe in critical thinking and evidence over acceptance or dogma; however, Peplau also pointed out that while people can heal in relationships, relationships can also contribute to human dysfunction.

In response to that cautious note, Reynolds (2000, 2009) suggested that nurses would be unable to facilitate satisfactory and productive outcomes for their clients unless they were able to empathize with accuracy.

Empathy and Therapeutic Outcomes

Kalkman (1967) states that relationship therapy enables the client to learn more satisfactory and productive patterns of behaviour. Several studies have supported the hypothesized relationship between empathy and favourable health outcomes. Achieving favourable health outcomes involves establishing needs, as determined by the client, and the resolution of problems.

Truax and Mitchell (1971) cite more than a dozen studies establishing that empathy is a major determinant of successful health outcomes for clients. Rogers (1975) summarized a sample of 22 research findings that supported his belief about the crucial role of the empathic process and improved health outcomes when the other person is 'hurting.'

Since Rogers' (1975) paper, the research evidence and claims in the theoretical literature has accumulated, and studies have supported the view that empathy is the primary ingredient in helping (therapeutic) relationships (e.g., Altman, 1983; Carver & Hughes, 1990; Gladstein, 1977; MacKay et al., 1990; Watson, 2014; Yu & Kirk, 2009).

While nursing research to date has only provided minimal evidence to support the view that clinical empathy in nursing affects therapeutic outcomes, the cumulative evidence across all helping professions indicates that the hypothesized relationship between empathy and helpful nurse–client relationships remains a reasonable proposition. The following studies encourage this view.

Williams (1979) studied the effects of empathy in the nursing care of institutionalized elderly to determine whether empathy might reduce the dehumanisation and depersonalisation of their environment, as measured by changes in self-concept. Nurses offered high and low levels of empathy to elderly clients over an eight-week period. A statistically significant increase in the self-concept of clients experiencing high empathy was demonstrated. Peplau (1990) suggests that adequate self-concept acts as an anti-anxiety device and results in more satisfactory relationships with significant others.

La Monica et al. (1987) explored the effect of nurses' empathy on anxiety, depression, and hostility in clients with cancer. They found less anxiety, depression, and hostility in clients being cared for by nurses exhibiting high empathy. More recent studies have continued to support the view that empathy is crucial to all helpful interpersonal relationships (e.g., Bove, 2019; Hardy, 2017; Lemmens et al., 2017; Murphy et al., 2018).

These findings indicate that there is a need for nursing to conduct more outcome studies in order to assess the relevance of empathy to clinical nursing. The urgency of that research agenda is indicated by the frequent reports of concerns about low empathy by professional helpers, including nurses.

Concerns about Low Empathy

While empathy is widely considered as critical to improving health care outcomes, several studies have indicated that many professional helpers, including nurses, are unable to offer empathy at a level necessary to understand the concerns of the client (Reynolds & Scott, 2000). The following examples illustrate this concern:

Hills and Knowles (1983) reported that nurses actually blocked clients' expressions by changing the subject, while Sloane (1993) reported that many physicians sampled in their study became defensive and withdrew from the client. Squire (1990) reported that a study of doctors' interpersonal skills demonstrated a tendency to dominate clinical interviews and ask for factual information, rather than listen to clients and reflect back on their feelings. More recently, Kitenge (2017) reported that nurses had negative attitudes towards HIV-positive clients, such as fear, anger, and frustration, which prevented nurses from offering empathy.

Williams (1992) pointed out that staff can experience crisis when they feel vulnerable, sad, and exposed during professional relationships, partly because they are experiencing aspects of life that are unfamiliar to them. This view is congruent with Kitenge's (2017) study, which reported that certain variables in clinical environments, as well as anxiety about competence, fear about health risks, and unsatisfactory support from work colleagues, resulted in nurses avoiding HIV-positive clients. Similarly, Reynolds (2000) reported that lack of time, lack of privacy, the clinical problems of clients, interruption to nurse–client conversations, and lack of support from unsympathetic colleagues negatively impacted nurse–patient relationships. Reynolds (2006) argued that barriers to empathy in clinical environments did not mean that empathy was not needed.

The culture and organization of the workplace can act as a disincentive to nurses' attempts to appreciate the client's perspective and respond in ways that result in favourable outcomes for those seeking help. Such organizational environments pose a problem because it is arguable that empathy is best learned in the workplace. Reynolds' (2000) study of empathy education showed that the most effective way of improving nurse's empathy was through supervised clinical practice involving process recordings of clinical interviews. Reynolds (2000) found that an experimental group of nurses made gains on all items on an empathy scale, while the control group of nurses did not make significant changes on any scale items, which led to the conclusion that when nurses are supported in the clinical environment, they are able to offer accurate empathy.

The Meaning and Components of Empathy

A limitation of the conclusions about available outcome studies is that empathy has been conceptualized and measured in different ways. It has been variously conceptualized as cognition, behaviour, a personality dimension, and an experienced emotion. The need to find a common definition of empathy is emphasized by the disagreement in the literature about what empathy means.

An extensive literature review by Morse et al. (1992) identified four components of empathy. These were: moral, emotive, cognitive, and behavioural. The moral component was identified as an internal altruistic force that motivates the practice of empathy. The emotive component was described as an ability to subjectively experience and share in another's psychological state or intrinsic feelings, which is sometimes referred to as sympathy. The cognitive component was defined as the helper's intellectual ability to identify and understand another person's feelings and perspective from an objective stance. Finally, the behavioural component was defined as a communicative response to convey understanding of another's perspective.

Similarly, Williams (1990) informs us that the most widely recognized components of empathy are emotional empathy, cognitive empathy, communicative empathy, and relational empathy. The additional component of relational empathy was defined as the experienced, or client-perceived empathy. This meant that empathy allows for the possibility of the client validating the helper's perception of their world. Williams' conclusion, which did not involve moral empathy, was broadly similar to Patterson's (1974) earlier definition of empathy.

Patterson (1974) described empathy as involving four concepts or stages. Firstly, the helper must be receptive to another's communication, the emotive or moral component. Secondly, the helper must understand the communication by putting himself in the other person's place, the cognitive component. Thirdly, the helper must communicate that understanding to the client, the behavioural or communicative component. Finally, Patterson suggested that empathy allowed for the possibility of the client to validate the helper's perception of the client's world, the relational component. The additional component of relational empathy is arguably an outcome that is dependent on and related to the helper's cognitive and behavioural ability so that the client may be offered the opportunity to validate the helper's perceptions and to experience being understood.

The different components of empathy identified by Morse et al. (1992) and others may all contribute to empathy, but the extent to which they are all interrelated appears to be a source of disagreement among theorists. This disagreement seems particularly emphasized in respect to what extent each component is applied or how they contribute to behaviours that build therapeutic problem-solving relationships. For example, it is possible that there needs to be fixed amounts of emotive empathy, or sympathy, in order to avoid interference with cognitive empathy. The relevance of emotive empathy to active listening is an interesting research problem.

Several theorists conceptualize empathy in a manner that emphasizes its cognitive-behavioural components. Thus, Truax (1961) wrote:

> Accurate empathy involves more than just the ability of the therapist to sense the client's private world as if it were his own. It also involves more than just the ability to know what the client means. Accurate empathy involves the sensitivity to current feelings and the verbal facility to communicate this understanding in a language attuned to the client's feelings.
>
> (p. 2)

The Truax definition emphasizes that empathy is a way of perceiving and communicating. It shifts the emphasis from a human trait to a form of interaction. This definition appears congruent with the cognitive and behavioural components of empathy alluded to by Morse et al. (1992).

Similarly, Rogers (1957), who tended to view empathy as an attitude, emphasized the communicative aspect of the construct. He suggested that the facilitative conditions operating in all effective relationships relate to the helper's attitude, cognition, and behaviour. Rogers argues that clients learn to change when helpers communicate warmth and genuineness and are successful in communicating understanding of clients' feelings. Later, Rogers (1975) repeated his view that the attitudes and cognitive ability of the helper are conveyed to the client through the communication of the helper. This view suggests that when attitudes and understanding are shown to the client, empathy is a skilled behaviour.

Rogers (1975) argues that warmth is a necessary condition that helps the client to change maladaptive coping responses to threats. He defines warmth as showing a commitment to helping and respect for the uniqueness of an individual. It seems reasonable to assume that showing commitment is likely to encourage a client to talk about sensitive issues, particularly if they feel respected. If the client is unable to talk about sensitive issues, accurate empathy is not possible. It is possible that warmth is similar to moral empathy and caring, since both concepts are concerned about the wellbeing of another.

Rogers (1975) also argues that genuineness is a critical condition for the development of therapeutic relationships. He stated that a genuine response meant that the counsellor was connected to their real self, a condition that Rogers called congruence, or authenticity. He also informs us that genuineness involves being direct, non-judgmental, and willing to be open about oneself. Rogers referred to that state as unconditional positive regard. Messages that are not direct (concrete) or are incompatible with the helper's self-image may prevent a trusting relationship from developing.

Truax and Carkhuff (1967) proposed that trust has its origins in warmth and genuineness and that these conditions are of central importance to any trusting relationship and have an interlocking nature with empathy. They pointed out that genuineness implies an openness to the experiences of the other person, a tendency to be non-judgmental.

Rogers (1961) states that an openness to the experiences of another involves listening to the feelings behind the words. However, he points out that a barrier to the exploration of feelings is the very natural tendency to judge, evaluate, or disapprove when a client's communication is ambiguous or personally threatening. He suggests that when this happens, helpers become defensive, often transmitting this defensiveness to the client through unwanted advice, failure to respond to direct questions, or curt, unfriendly voice tone (Rogers, 1961). Kitenge (2017) offered an example of this tendency when he reported that nurses' attitudes, such as fear, anger, and frustration towards HIV-positive clients prevented them from offering warmth and genuineness to their clients. Rogers and Truax (1967) proposed that the logical means of correcting this tendency is to work on achieving genuineness. They suggest that once this is established, the work of helping proceeds through the helper's moment-by-moment empathic grasp of the significance of the client's world.

The Measurement of Empathy

While there is a need for nurses to know when they are offering empathy, challenges to the measurement of empathy relate to the confusion about what empathy means (Reynolds, 1987). Reynolds (2000) developed a measure of cognitive-behavioural empathy that reflected clients' perceptions of being understood by nurses. A concern about the existing measures of cognitive-behavioural empathy was that the client's perception of the helping relationship was not reflected during construction of the tool. Clients' perceptions of their relationship with nurses helped to clarify the meaning of empathy in nursing. The Reynolds Empathy Scale (RES) was comprised of 12 items, with six items that measured what clients wanted in the relationship and six items that measured what they did not want.

What clients wanted from a nurse:

- Attempts to explore and clarify feelings
- Responds to feelings
- Explores personal meaning of feelings
- Responds to feelings and meanings
- Provides the client with direction that assists the client to find solutions that reflect their preferences
- Appropriate voice tone, sounds relaxed.

What clients did not want from a nurse:

- Leads, directs, and diverts
- Ignores verbal and non-verbal communication
- Judgmental and opinionated
- Interrupts and seems in a hurry
- Fails to focus on solutions/does not answer direct questions/lacks genuineness
- Inappropriate voice tone, sounds curt.

A study by Mercer and Reynolds (2002) confirmed the scale's reliability and construct validity. Gosselin et al. (2015) investigated the validity of a French version of the RES. They reported that the scale had good inter-rater reliability and good psychometric properties. The RES has now been utilized as a research and teaching tool in several other countries including Spain, Finland, Taiwan, Iran, the USA, and Swaziland.

9 New Technologies

Kamini Kalia and Amy Lewis

Digital health technologies serve to support, enable, as well as ameliorate healthcare workflow practices; increase access to information; and provide central functions for optimal healthcare delivery and partnership between clients and clinicians. Thoughtful consideration regarding the use of technology to deliver healthcare is essential, as shifts to the traditional therapeutic relationship may occur. Despite emerging research that suggests technology integration provides comparable clinical outcomes for a variety of illnesses, skepticism exists regarding their impact on client safety, the therapeutic relationship, and quality of care (Barrett & Gershkovich, 2014; Manfrida et al., 2017; Schuster et al., 2018). This chapter explores digital health technologies and their integration within the therapeutic relationship, followed by clinical considerations for using digital health technologies.

Digital Health Technologies

The World Health Organization (2020) defines eHealth as "the use of information and communication technologies for health" (para. 1). This broad definition covers a spectrum of technical and therapeutic modalities. For the purpose of this chapter, eHealth will be used interchangeably with other terms that describe physical or psychological interventions offered through a technical modality, including e-therapy, telehealth, telemedicine, telepsychiatry, telepsychology, videoconferencing, Internet-based therapy, psychotherapeutic interventions, and mHealth (mobile mental health).

The Digital Therapeutic Relationship

The therapeutic relationship is central for successful face-to-face clinical outcomes, and in particular, for psychotherapy (Lambert & Barley, 2001; Norcross & Wampold, 2011). The traditional therapeutic relationship may be best illustrated as recurring, in-person clinical visits in a structured physical environment, such as an office or client's home. The digital therapeutic relationship expands the possibility for interaction by leveraging technology to improve access to care. In this experience, the environment goes beyond the traditional physical office or home to wherever the client and device are situated. Similarly, the clinician's availability and engagement may be more frequent, dynamic, and less structured.

Clinicians can take advantage of the plethora of mobile health technologies via the therapeutic relationship. For instance, clients can electronically track health data (e.g., activity levels, quantity and quality of sleep, and degree of social interaction) that are entered into algorithms that predict clinical outcomes and alert the clinician to revise the care plan and strengthen clients' self-management of a chronic condition (IQVIA Institute, 2017). There is significant potential for precision and personalized interventions based on the data collated from digital health apps and programs. This model of care can help manage exacerbations of illness that otherwise burden acute care services. When used to support the therapeutic relationship, digital health technologies can increase collaboration and trust, as well as support clients in managing their illness.

Despite research supporting that the quality of the therapeutic relationship is predictive of clinical outcomes, fears exist with using digital technology to support the therapeutic relationship, including risk to client care, legal issues, ethics, treatment fidelity and efficacy, workload, technology glitches, authenticity, and existing jobs (Manfrida et al., 2017; Richards et al., 2018; Torous & Hsin, 2018). Similar to other treatment modalities, such as medications or surgery, the benefits of a particular service come with unintentional risks that clinicians must be aware of prior to use. Considerations regarding digital health technology will now be discussed.

Common Considerations for Digital Health Technology Use

Goals of Therapy

Agreement between the client and clinician regarding the goals of treatment is foundational to the relationship, so the use of digital health technology should be outlined by the clinician before the service starts (Morris & Aguilera, 2012). Clinicians can determine the suitability of using technology by exploring the client's experience, comfort of use, and technical needs. As the therapeutic relationship progresses, it is important for the clinician to review this alignment with established and changing treatment goals and expectations (Roberts & Torous, 2017).

Clinician Competencies

Clinician Attitudes and Behaviours

Clinicians agree upon the importance of the therapeutic relationship; however, clinicians report decreased confidence in their ability to establish an alliance by e-therapy compared to in-person interactions (Sucala et al., 2013). Clinician training is necessary to increase confidence, shift attitudes, and prevent barriers to developing digital therapeutic relationships. General topics to consider include privacy and confidentiality, consent, therapeutic boundaries, ethics, crisis management, and risk mitigation. Cultural competence is an important topic if remote services are provided outside of one's own culture (Henry et al., 2017; Quackenbush & Krasner, 2012). Communication styles, cultural nuances, cultural values and belief systems, health and illness education, stigma, and family systems may be conveyed differently through a virtual medium. Furthermore, relevant legal and regulatory requirements and obligations (e.g., documentation and data collection) should be reviewed as it applies to the digital context (Reamer, 2015; Schuster et al., 2018). Clinicians should be familiar with regional legislation where they are licensed to provide care and maintain appropriate insurance coverage (Reamer, 2015). In addition, it is valuable to have a basic understanding of relevant and reliable evaluation tools to assess outcomes, progress, and quality of care using digital health technologies to determine the effectiveness of service delivery.

Technological Skills

Clinicians need an adequate understanding of digital clinical tools to effectively communicate with clients and provide troubleshooting support, if necessary (Reamer, 2015). It is important that clinicians assess the technical abilities, digital literacy, and health information literacy of clients and to consider time constraints involved with using technology (Canadian Internet Registration Authority [CIRA], 2018; Ho & Quick, 2018; Williams et al., 2018). Clinicians can collaborate with clients to address technical competencies for successful adoption.

Therapeutic Environment

Similar to in-person treatment, the digital therapeutic environment must be supportive to clients when provided online. Clinicians can proactively address potential risks to the client in regard to their own environment, as they have less control online (Henry et al., 2017). Environmental factors to consider include proper lighting, managing distractions, limiting the number of participants, and preventing potential interruptions. Privacy issues can be addressed by using headphones, having familiarity with technical equipment, and using a private area (Henry et al., 2017; Strudwick et al., 2019; Wade et al., 2019).

Conscious Communication Skills

Henry et al. (2017) conducted a systematic review on telehealth care delivery that revealed verbal communication as an important dynamic in the therapeutic relationship. Telehealth verbal communications have been criticized for being perceived as more focused on tasks and getting to the matter at hand, while being less attentive to important social nuances, for instance, the expression of clinician empathy (Henry et al., 2017). Non-verbal communication, such as facial gestures, tone of voice, eye contact, and body movement, is another critical element to the development and maintenance of trust – the basis of the digital therapeutic relationship (DeLucia et al., 2013; Manfrida et al., 2017; Wade et al., 2019). Evidence from multiple systematic reviews highlights the importance of considering how non-verbal cues are expressed online, for example, through visible physical gestures; overemphasizing one's actions, such as nodding or facial expressions; demonstrating attentiveness; and ensuring good visual view of the clinician and their body language (DeLucia et al., 2013; Henry et al., 2017).

Email is typically used to replace face-to-face sessions; however, the length of the communication and less frequent nature of emails may impact the impression of the clinician and the timeliness of the issue compared to instant messaging or short message service (SMS) conversational communications. Manfrida et al. (2017) describe online communication as a mechanism to support open communication within the context of a therapeutic relationship. Maintaining open communication online means addressing the time limits of traditional therapy, reassuring clients regarding clinician availability, reducing the frequency and cost of sessions, and helping clinicians to effectively manage their autonomy in terms of how and when they may respond to communications (Manfrida et al., 2017). Open, online communication also extends clinical interventions beyond the session to allow clinicians to further decode the meaning of the message, in other words, clinicians have more time to review the email communications from clients before they respond.

Manfrida et al. (2017) also explain that SMS has been overthrown by instant messaging (e.g., WhatsApp) in more recent years. Although instant messaging has become more common than SMS messaging, the informal nature of this application presents a potential risk for clinicians. Internet-based messaging tends to involve a more casual communication, stylistic, or punctuation nuances; an increased quantity of messages sent and received; use of emojis or emoticons (images via text) to convey emotions or thoughts; and potentially, conveyance of personal information, such as profile photographs, location, and more, depending on what is depicted in photos. Clinicians should exercise some level of caution and professionalism when using these technologies to maintain a therapeutic versus social relationship. In addition, instant messaging applications collect and make available information to its users on user-availability and when messages were sent and reviewed, while also relying on Wi-Fi connection for the delivery and retrieval of messages (DeLucia et al, 2013). WhatsApp has the option to create group chats, which can be helpful to communicate to groups of people, such as multiple clinicians who are participating in one chat (Manfrida et al., 2017). Some of these features can be turned off, but if they are not, professional boundaries of engagement must be exercised. Setting boundaries includes communicating expectations of using this technology to clients, involving another clinician to manage communications, and limiting engagement to particular hours of the day.

Preventing Harm and Mitigating Risks

Clinicians who use digital technologies in their work must be diligent and responsible to ensure the same degree of safety is exercised as in-person services (Roberts & Torous, 2017; Torous & Hsin, 2018). Torous and Roberts (2017) introduced an ethical framework to mitigate potential risks of technologies that target vulnerable populations, cause unanticipated harm, make false or unsubstantiated claims, or whereby the role or responsibility of clinicians has yet to be established. The ethical framework includes a review of the benefits and risks of introducing the mobile technology into care. A conscious effort to trial and evaluate technologies prior to their use is important, as the validity, effectiveness, and safety of these technologies are still under investigation. Given the newness of some of these technologies, clinical supervision may also support a clinician who is eager to integrate these tools into clinical practice (Reamer, 2015).

Informed Consent and Privacy

Informed consent must be obtained, followed by a discussion of client confidentiality concerns (i.e., there may be no guarantee of a privacy policy with particular apps; potential for privacy breach). Clinicians must manage the obligation of maintaining confidentiality with the client's choice of software. In some ways, there is increased accessibility in that the consumer can select or purchase applications with this business model; however, this may be in conflict with the ethics of the therapeutic relationship (Torous & Roberts, 2017). In other words, the security and privacy of the client must be maintained, but this may be in conflict with the industry who is collecting this data (Reamer, 2015; Torous & Roberts, 2017).

Policies and Guidelines

Within clinical settings, employers can institute social media or telemedicine policies that provide guidelines and establish safeguards to prevent harm and enhance adherence to legal requirements, practice regulations, or other interdependent policies and procedures (Reamer, 2015). These supports may preserve privacy and confidentiality by implementing measures to prevent a clinician from sending an email or text to the wrong recipient (Reamer, 2015).

Licensing and Scope of Practice

It is in the best interest of all those involved for clinicians to prevent lawsuits and regulatory and licensing complaints, while mitigating risks and preventing harm to clients (Reamer, 2015). Clinicians should possess a valid licence and insurance to practice over the Internet and consider issues related to scope of practice. One example of a scope of practice concern relates to legal acts, such as the provision of psychotherapy in Ontario, Canada (Mental Health Commission of Canada [MHCC], 2014). Clinicians who are not regulated to initiate or perform controlled acts of psychotherapy may alter language (e.g., from "psychotherapy" to "education" or "coaching"), thus bypassing the regulation that is in place to protect the public.

Additional questions to review in terms of ethics include:

- Should the digital health technology be available as an adjunct to or a replacement for therapy/treatment?
- Why has the particular technology been selected for use? Is the technology consumer-driven or market-driven?
- How will consent, privacy, and confidentiality be addressed?
- How can risk be minimized for vulnerable populations?
- Is the technology safe for a client to use without guidance from or direct access to a clinician?
- What is the availability of the clinician?
- How will emergencies or crises be managed?
- When will the therapeutic relationship terminate and how does this occur?

Clinician Roles

With shifts in access to information, consumer-driven technologies and their demand, and power dynamics, the roles of the clinician may be questioned and adapted (Schuster et al., 2018). It is imperative that clinicians embrace the role of educator and broker of health information, particularly when information on the Internet is becoming increasingly accessible and prolific in fake or inaccurate information, which is sometimes targeted to the consumer using commercial algorithms. Concerns regarding the accuracy and validity of various applications and information come into question and can exacerbate anxiety (Ho & Quick, 2018). Clinicians can efficiently sift through credible and reliable sources of health information, or even create health resources.

With the use of wearable and mobile monitoring devices, the focus of the therapeutic relationship can shift to the topic of genetic or nutritional counseling (MHCC, 2014). Eventually, digital health technology may help clinicians, and even clients, determine the type of modality required for therapy based on diagnosis or other variables. The dynamic nature of clinician roles continues to exist in digital health technologies where the clinician role may shift into a teacher or coaching role for milder illnesses, and then a surrogate role for more severe stages of illness or complex cases (MHCC, 2014). Considerations regarding how to leverage technologies to maximize a workforce are encouraged. For example, in the case of "low intensity interventions," which refer to the delivery of services that do not require specific expertise or training, a broader mental health workforce may be able to offer services and increase the accessibility of standard care (Thomas et al., 2016), freeing up clinical expertise to manage more severe and complex cases.

Information Development and Exchange

Self-help programs are very cost-effective as they do not require a clinician or facilitator. Although effective, these programs lack individualization (Schuster et al., 2018). Many self-monitoring apps and devices are also available "direct to consumer" (Ho & Quick, 2018), which may put a strain on the therapeutic relationship if the clinician is not in support of the technology. Clinicians, credible bodies, and authors of systematic reviews have evaluated some of the existing apps and made their assessments available online (MHCC, 2014). Portals like http://beacon.anu.edu.au/ provide information that is categorized by illness. Knowledge hubs, developed by clients, clinicians, and caregivers, also enable credible information about evidence-based treatments to be more accessible to the public.

Addressing Access

Despite the trend of ubiquitous mobile technology, marginalized communities are still disadvantaged in terms of access to the Internet, including adults aged 75 and up, Indigenous Peoples, and individuals living in remote and rural communities (Anderson & Perrin, 2017; CIRA, 2018). The health of the client may also impact their ability to select and use a technology. For example, individuals who have limitations in executive functioning, motor control, and concentration may experience challenges while using technology, which can limit their access to virtual healthcare. Further work is needed by policymakers, funding agencies, and advocates to reach these populations so they too can benefit from technological innovations to address these inequities (CIRA, 2018).

Poor connectivity and technical challenges have reportedly impacted clients' perceived satisfaction with technology, thus creating a barrier to use (Jenkins-Guarnieri et al., 2015). Clinicians should first review whether the individual has access to troubleshooting support, hardware that is in good working condition, and reliable connectivity. Similarly, researchers and their collaborators also need to consider how research participants will have access to digital technology post-study (Torous & Hsin, 2018).

Conclusion

There is an array of technology and tools available to support and transform healthcare delivery. Some technologies are relevant and closely tied to the therapeutic relationship, such as videoconferencing, while others are not, like self-management health tools with personalized prompts. These digital health technologies may not replace the traditional therapeutic relationship but do offer a better standard than a waitlist and can reduce burden on acute care services. Although several benefits exist around the use of digital health technologies, some important considerations must be addressed before digital health technologies are integrated within clinical work.

10 Ethics and Boundaries in Therapeutic Relationships

Brad A. MacNeil, Cheryl Forchuk, and Abraham Rudnick

Mental healthcare is rife with ethics issues. Matters of access, coercion, confidentiality, therapeutic boundaries and more are particularly prominent in mental healthcare. Transitional mental healthcare typically involves time-limited mental healthcare to bridge services, e.g., between inpatient and outpatient services; yet, not much has been published about transitional mental healthcare ethics. Indeed, even in what may be the most studied part of transitional mental healthcare ethics, i.e., ethics of transition of mental healthcare from childhood to adulthood, very little has been published, and much, if not all of it, is not conceptually robust or not methodologically rigorous (Paul et al., 2018).

Transitional Mental Healthcare Ethics

Transitional mental healthcare addresses various clinical populations and their differing needs. For example, it addresses the transition of service users from child mental health services to adult mental health services, from adult mental health services to senior mental health services, from inpatient mental health services to outpatient mental health services, and from one individual service provider to another individual service provider within the same service (Jayaram, 2015).

Ethics refers to conflict or tension between moral values and to reasoned approaches that attempt to resolve such conflict or tension in a publicly acceptable manner. In healthcare, recent and current ethics commonly address conflict or tension between the values of autonomy (or self-determination of service users), beneficence (or best interests of service users), non-maleficence (or doing least harm to service users while providing them healthcare), and justice (or equity for all people in need of health services rather than for some but not others) (Beauchamp & Childress, 2012). Dialogical ethics, on the other hand, prioritizes the process rather than the content of communication between the involved parties in relevant healthcare situations (Rudnick, 2001, 2002).

Mental healthcare ethics address issues that arise exclusively or prominently in mental healthcare. Examples include lack of access to evidence-based psychotherapy and society's coercion of many people with mental health challenges. Confidentiality is important to address in mental healthcare as it often involves particularly sensitive personal information, sometimes about third parties, such as service users' families. Critical reasoning to achieve an acceptable balance of values, such as autonomy, beneficence, non-maleficence, and justice, is helpful to resolve ethics challenges (Rudnick, 2019). For example, equitable access to psychotherapy should be promoted as much as possible without considerably compromising access to other important services for the public. Coercion of people with mental health challenges should be minimized so that it is reserved for life threatening situations. And confidentiality of service users' mental health information should be breached only if not doing so poses a considerable safety risk.

Another ethics issue of transitional mental healthcare is multiplicity of mental healthcare providers involved with service users' care, creating potential communication and service challenges thus possibly compromising safety (Jayaram, 2015). It may help therapeutic relationships to use demonstrated safeguards, such as standardized processes of communication and associated protocols, and related education for service users and their providers (Buckman, 2010).

Therapeutic Boundaries in Transitional Mental Healthcare

Transitional mental healthcare involves the careful coordination of services across organizational policy, programs, and individual service providers aimed at ensuring the continuity of care for service users from one care episode to the next (Coleman & Berenson, 2004). Although providers routinely approach these care transition points with the best intentions, transition points in a service user's journey through the mental health and addictions system may represent periods of increased vulnerability for professional boundary transgressions.

The delivery of mental healthcare comes with a fiduciary obligation of healthcare organizations and providers to act in the best interests of service users (Kutchins, 1991). There is an inherent power differential in this relationship, as the provider knows much more about the service user than the service user knows about the provider (and knowledge is power). Boundaries refer to the social, emotional, psychological, and physical space between a service provider and a service user (Strohm-Kitchener & Anderson, 2011). When considering the elements of professional boundaries, it is important to distinguish between boundary crossings, boundary violations (both sometimes termed boundary transgressions), and egregious boundary transgressions such as sexual misconduct (Peternelj-Taylor & Young, 2003).

Boundary crossings are characterized as a divergence from the formal act of providing service to a service user (Gutheil & Simon, 2002). Gutheil and Gabbard (1993) argued that the line is crossed when the service provider steps into a non-therapeutic or non-clinical role with the service user. It may be a temporary change in the status of the formal therapeutic relationship whereby the service provider draws personal benefit in some way from the interaction.

Reamer (2003) categorized boundary crossings into specific domains that encompass some transition points of care, including those that involve personal gain (e.g., financial), emotional needs (e.g., a service provider reversing roles with a service user they provide service to), philanthropic gestures (e.g., offering favors and gift giving), and unforeseen situations (e.g., informal meetings at local events or having mutual connections). Other examples of boundary crossings in transitional mental health and addictions services include some forms of unnecessary self-disclosure, extending the length of service past what is required, providing unlimited availability to a service user, interacting on social media platforms outside of care, and physical contact and intimacy (Gutheil & Simon, 1995). Vulnerability for some of these boundary crossings may be heightened at transition points in care. Transitioning a service user to a new provider or ending an episode of care raises the chances being confronted with a thank you gift, the space for unnecessary self-disclosure, or pressure (either internal to the provider or external by the service user) to extend the length of care. Context also plays a role. Research has shown that professionals practicing in rural areas differ in their views on boundary crossings that may make the line between formal and less professional dual roles more difficult to distinguish (Borys & Pope, 1989); it is not uncommon in rural communities for the service provider to have to provide care to a neighbor as there is no other provider available: Note that providing service to a family member is particularly problematic and should be avoided. A recent review of the literature revealed common aspects of individuals who engage in boundary crossings, including engaging in dual relationships, accepting or exchanging of gifts with service users, engagement in secret behaviour, overinvolvement, social media use, and physical contact (Manfrin-Ledet et al., 2015).

Boundaries during transitions also require some flexibility as providers and service users have lives outside of the formal service delivery and organizations where services occur, which may intersect with providers' professional identity. Such situations may include unexpectedly meeting service users at a restaurant or grocery store, having their children attend the same school or activity programming, and sharing a peer group (Austin et al., 2006). The interpersonal qualities that make service providers effective in their roles may also make them more vulnerable to the slippery slope of relaxing boundaries leading to escalating boundary violations (Anderson & Handelsman, 2010). Transition points in care may raise a service provider's vulnerability for relaxing professional boundaries in an attempt to cope with their own emotional reaction to the transition.

The transition time between the end of the intentional therapy session and the client moving to the office door is a brief time when both service user and service provider are at greater vulnerability (Gutheil & Simon, 1995). A provider may experience a sense of accomplishment after ending an episode of care where a service user has met their care plan goals or experience a sense of self-doubt when a service user does not. Transition points in mental healthcare also represent times when providers are required to pick up new service users on their caseloads. A provider's experiences at the time of ending the therapeutic relationship is one variable that has not received much attention in the literature. One study showed that social workers and social work trainees endorsed that it is generally difficult to end an episode of care and viewed it as especially adverse with accompanying negative emotions when care is ended by the service user themselves (Baum, 2007).

Steadman (1992) described so-called boundary spanners as a factor associated with greater efficacy in programs, representing a role in which service providers span services across competing systems (e.g., corrections, mental healthcare, and more) through the use of specialized and generic skillsets. Errors in the provision of services at the system level may also be heightened at this transition time. This risk is especially true during transitions from inpatient to outpatient care, which have generally documented that errors occur in approximately half of transitions and are associated with a higher risk for service users to be readmitted (Moore et al., 2003). Errors with not receiving the proper service user consent for sharing information with the new organization or provider, as well as errors with not following through on the uptake of the new service by the service user, may be common at these transitions.

Interprofessional perspectives on professionalism (i.e., acceptable conduct) during interactions with service users at transitional points in care may vary across disciplines and settings within mental healthcare. For example, having coffee with a service user as part of community-based recovery coaching may be widely acceptable; however, having coffee in the community with a service user would represent a boundary violation for a therapist in another context, such as exploratory/expressive psychotherapy. Professional standards also evolve and change over the career trajectory of healthcare providers (Wagner et al., 2007). For example, research has shown that some professionals are at greater risk of boundary crossings early in their careers (Baca, 2009).

Community-based recovery coaches or system navigators may have the opportunity to interact formally with service users during the provision of care in a number of informal settings and at various transition points. These settings may include coffee shops, hospital cafeteria, local parks, grocery stores, and the service users' home. Day-to-day interactions tend to be less structured and formal in community-based practice compared to conventional psychotherapy. Transition points may also be viewed as less formal and leave an opportunity for boundary crossings to emerge. The casual nature as perceived by the service user may make the development and maintenance of professional boundaries in these relationships challenging; some have argued that if community-based recovery coaches are not routinely facing boundary issues in their work, they may be providing less effective care (Curtis & Hodge, 1994).

Although boundary crossings may begin as quite harmless in nature, and may even support the process of service provision, they may become more progressive and evolve into boundary violations over time (Gutheil & Simon, 2002). Garfinkel and colleagues (1997) described the therapeutic relationship as a unique context where emotional responses are induced, and the service provider may be more likely to act on those strong emotions with service users. Characteristics considered to be predictors of boundary violations by service providers have been categorized by Barnett (2014) into individual differences (e.g., personality factors), unskillfulness (e.g., skills deficits related to handling challenging service users), and situational (e.g., service providers experiencing personal stressors). Boundary violations represent a harmful or possibly damaging informal interaction that occurs within the context of service provision and results in the exploitation of the service user (Gutheil & Simon, 2002).

Intimate and sexual relationships between service providers and users have received much empirical attention due to the destructive nature of these boundary violations. Sexual contact with service users among service providers in healthcare ranges from 3% to 12% (Berkman et al., 2000). Research has shown that 1% of mental healthcare providers endorsed having had sexual contact with a current or former service user (Borys & Pope, 1989). Engagement in antisocial behaviour, being male, working in private practice, having undergone their own psychotherapy (indicating a mental health challenge rather than the disruptive effect of receiving psychotherapy on service providers), and having a defensive style have been associated with these types of boundary violations and eventual revocation of a professional license (Garfinkel et al., 1997).

With a boundary violation, the actions of the service provider harm the service user (Epstein, 1994). Boundary crossings, by comparison, are dual relationships that are not intentionally exploitative or expected to be so, and therefore may not be inherently unethical (Reamer, 2003), although unintended but foreseeable consequences should be expected and avoided as much as possible.

The vulnerability for professionals to experience boundary drift within the social media platform is different from real world interactions due to factors including social media's deindividuation, the speed of communication, the lack of clear hierarchy, and power differentials (Cooper & Inglehearn, 2015). Part of this is due to the integration of multiple contexts and audiences that create challenges for professionals on social media platforms (Marwick & Boyd, 2010). These audiences may range from service users, to families and friends of service users, to other care providers, to the various levels at organizations.

Education and self-reflection on boundaries, boundary crossings, and boundary violations are an important part of transitional care and ongoing professional development. Transitional care that centres on the fiduciary responsibility of organizations and providers, as well as the safety and trust of the service user, are also important in this regard. Service providers also need to make choices based on their moral responsibility, with the service users' best interests kept in mind during transitions in care (Black, 2017).

Conclusion

Ethical practice and understanding the nature of professional boundaries is essential to all mental healthcare. However, the period of transitioning services is a time when roles are in flux and therefore boundaries may be vulnerable. Self-reflection, education, and clear policies assist in maintaining ethical practices.

Part V

From Therapeutic Relationships to Transitional Care

This section of the book moves from considering therapeutic relationships to considering transitional care. In particular, this section highlights the development, implementation, and testing of the transitional discharge model (TDM).

The TDM was developed shortly after I completed my PhD in 1992. Seven weeks after I defended my PhD, my youngest daughter was born, and I was on maternity leave for most of the year. Upon returning to Hamilton Psychiatric Hospital, the suggestion was that I move to a different part of the schizophrenia program due to problems with discharge on that particular inpatient unit. The hospital was a provincial psychiatric hospital that provided tertiary care where people typically had a couple of admissions to a general hospital psychiatric unit (secondary level care) but required more specialized care. The length of stay in our facility was the shortest of all the tertiary care provincial hospitals in Ontario, Canada at that time. The average length of stay was only 21 days, which was less than some secondary care facilities. Lengths of stay ranged depending on program; however, we had one unit that was clearly an outlier. To get to this program, people had to have had five years of hospitalization. Although the program was supposed to be for 25 people, few people left, so the census swelled to 38, which meant that no private rooms were available, and the unit was crowded and noisy. In the previous year, clients had a better chance of getting off the ward by death (3 people) than by discharge (2 people). I agreed to work on this unit if we could involve all the clients and staff on the ward in a participatory action project. I received assurances from hospital leadership that we could implement whatever was suggested.

I started the project by having weekly meetings with staff and clients to look at issues related to discharge. The minutes from these meetings were available to both groups. A central steering committee was composed of staff, clients on the ward, and people who had successfully left the ward and were living in the community. Staff and clients nominated their members to form this group. These minutes were also available to staff and clients.

People on the ward were initially reluctant to discuss leaving the hospital, and we agreed to involve a newly formed community group of psychiatric consumer-survivors (people with the experience of psychiatric illness). (This group later evolved into the Mental Health Rights Coalition [MHRC] of Hamilton group, and received provincial funding.) A critical meeting was facilitated by a former client and members of that group without staff presence. (Matthew Sircilj, who was a co-author on the pilot papers emerging from this work, played this key role; he was assisted that day by Susan Roach who became director of MHRC and later of a similar group in Simcoe, Ontario.) People who were living on the unit identified the importance of relationships to the transition from hospital to the community. They said that the unit had become home and that staff and fellow clients were like friends and family. They felt like they had no one to support them outside of the hospital. Their challenge to us was: come up with a way to have supportive relationships in the community and they would happily leave.

In the interest of space, I will not go into all of the details, but that advisory group worked very hard on this goal. Nurse manager Tessie Valledor, staff nurse Jackie Jewell, and clinical nurse specialist Mary-Lou Martin represented some of the staff in the advisory group. We partnered with a mental health team from public health that followed people after discharge, including Vicki Woodcox, Ruth Schofield, and Barb Overby. Other than Matthew Sircilj, client representatives chose not to be named publicly.

The new model had two critical components: (a) staff would continue to see people leaving the hospital until a therapeutic relationship was established in the community. This involved a three-way consensus: the hospital staff, community staff, and client all had to agree that a therapeutic relationship was established; and (b) people leaving the hospital would receive peer support from someone who had a previous experience of mental illness and who was now living in the community. Peer support can take many forms, but this was a friendship model of peer support.

The program was very successful and in the year it was implemented 13 people were discharged with only two very brief (less than two weeks) readmissions. No new funding was provided to allow staff to see people post-discharge; however, we reallocated resources so that for every two people discharged, we reduced the available "beds" by one until we reached the more manageable census of 25. A summary of the results from the first year of this project, including a cost analysis, was published as Forchuk, Chan, et al. (1998) "Bridging the Discharge Process." The phrase "bridging" was inspired by people on the unit who drew pictures of what the model should look like, with drawings frequently featuring "bridges," and from discussions that those bridges represented people who would help. Other papers form the pilot project include qualitative feedback from staff and clients (Forchuk, Schofield, et al., 1998), a theoretical discussion of the process relating the model as an extension of Peplau's theory to a broader interprofessional approach (Forchuk, Jewell, et al., 1998), and a paper outlining how we promoted independent living post-discharge (Schofield et al., 1997). Notably, all 38 people on the unit at the start of the pilot project were successfully discharged.

The pilot unit was an unusual one with very long lengths of stay (years). We then had a project to look at implementing the model on a variety of inpatient units in four different provincial psychiatric hospitals. Thirteen units were matched with 13 similar units. Matching included clinical focus (for example, forensic programs matched with forensic programs, adolescent programs with adolescent programs, mood programs with mood programs, etc.) and average length of stay as a proxy for chronicity. Over 40 units volunteered but we could only involve 26 that had reasonable matches. The results of this project are included as Chapter 11, "Therapeutic Relationships: From Psychiatric Hospital to Community" by Cheryl Forchuk, Mary-Lou Martin, Yee-Ching (Lilian) Chan, and Elsabeth Jensen [previously published as Forchuk, C., Martin, M.-L., Chan, L., & Jensen, E. (2005). Therapeutic relationships: From psychiatric hospital to community. *Journal of Psychiatric and Mental Health Nursing, 12*(5), 556–564. https://doi.org/10.1111/j.1365-2850.2005.00873.x]. This chapter took the TDM developed in the pilot and tested it with a wider number of psychiatric wards. Within the 13 pairs of wards, one ward was randomized to the TDM, while the other ward continued with usual care. Although the wards were matched for clinical focus and similar lengths of stay, the intervention wards after implementation discharged patients 124 days faster, with slightly fewer readmissions.

Over the years, we have implemented and tested this model in different programs and countries. Recently in Ontario, Canada, the Council of Academic Hospitals of Ontario (CAHO) declared the TDM a best practice based on consistent findings of reduced length of stay and lower hospital readmissions. They also gave us funding to implement it in nine Ontario hospitals with acute care programs (secondary level care – usually first and second admissions) as well as tertiary care programs.

Chapter 12 entitled, "Peer Support," which is an important part of transitional discharge, written by Cheryl Forchuk, Michelle Solomon, and Tazim Virani [previously published as Forchuk, C., Solomon, M., & Virani, T. (2016). Peer support: An important part of transitional discharge. *Healthcare Quarterly*, *18*(special issue), 32–36. https://doi.org/10.12927/hcq.2016 .24480], focuses on findings from peer support networks in Southwestern Ontario. The experience of CONNECT for Mental Health in providing peer support during the CAHO project is highlighted. Chapter 13 is a summary of focus group findings from different stakeholder groups during the CAHO project. This chapter is entitled "Implementation of a Transitional Discharge Model: Clients, Health Professionals, and Peer Supporters' Perspectives" written by Boniface Harerimana, Sebastian Gyamfi, and Cheryl Forchuk.

Chapter 14, "Cost-Effectiveness of the Implementation of a Transitional Discharge Model for Community Integration of Psychiatric Clients: Practice Insights and Policy Implications," authored by Cheryl Forchuk, Mary-Lou Martin, Deborah Corring, Deborrah Sherman, Rani Srivastava, Boniface Harerimana, and Raymond Cheng [previously published as Forchuk, C., Martin, M.-L., Corring, D., Sherman, D., Srivastava, R., Harerimana, B., & Cheng, R. (2019). Cost-effectiveness of the implementation of a transitional discharge model for community integration of psychiatric clients: Practice insights and policy implications. *International Journal of Mental Health*, *48*(3), 236–249. https://doi.org/10.1080/00207411.2019.1649237], outlines cost-savings and policy considerations from the CAHO project. This topic is similar to Chapter 11 in that both look at costs; however, Chapter 11 only looked at tertiary care units that had comparatively longer lengths of stay. The difference of 124 days between the intervention and control units relate to the tertiary nature of the wards. In Chapter 14, acute care units with much shorter lengths of stay are included. Therefore, the reduction in length of stay is also shorter but since there are far more discharges from acute care units, the cost-savings is actually greater.

Chapter 15 is written by Mary-Lou Martin who has been involved in numerous studies related to the TDM, including the pilot phase. This chapter is entitled "Supporting Therapeutic Relationships in the Clinical Setting." It outlines policies and practices that can be used to support therapeutic relationships in hospital and clinical community settings.

Finally, Chapter 16 is the "Conclusion" written by myself, Cheryl Forchuk. This chapter summarizes the journey and work on therapeutic relationships and transitional care. Note that after the conclusion, the appendices include toolkit items that were helpful for programs implementing the TDM.

11 Therapeutic Relationships

From Psychiatric Hospital to Community

Cheryl Forchuk, Mary-Lou Martin, Yee-Ching (Lilian) Chan, and Elsabeth Jensen

The mental healthcare system is in the midst of continued change and reform in the province of Ontario, Canada. The number of psychiatric hospital beds is being dramatically reduced and the emphasis is on service provision in the community. This pattern is similar to other jurisdictions. For example, it is reported that in the USA the number of long-stay occupied beds decreased by 50% between 1991 and 1997 (Desai & Rosenheck, 2003). The transition from hospital to community is complex and can be challenging for individual clients. A recent study of 85 long-term patients showed that 25% met the criterion for relocation trauma when moved from hospital to community (Farhall et al., 2003). In order to successfully move the focus of care to the community, effective models of care are required.

Transitional Discharge Model (TDM)

From 1993 to 1996, a pilot project called "Bridge to Discharge" took place on a tertiary care ward in which care was provided to individuals diagnosed with schizophrenia who had been hospitalized for a minimum of five years. Prior to the implementation of the pilot, few clients were successfully returned to the community. Data provided from the clinical records department of the hospital revealed that in the five years prior to the pilot, discharges ranged from one to four patients annually. The average census increased from 30 to 38 clients over this five-year period (1988–1993). The pilot study involved clients, staff, a community mental health program, a consumer-survivor group, and researchers in the process of developing strategies for successful transition to the community. A transitional discharge model (TDM) was developed based on a safety net of professional and peer relationships (Forchuk, Jewell, et al., 1998). The TDM builds on Peplau's interpersonal theory of nursing (Peplau, 1991). It assumes that the quality of interpersonal relationships has an influence and impact on quality of life and that a supportive social network will promote less need for expensive interventions such as hospitalization. This TDM had two components: (a) inpatient staff who continued to care for discharged clients until therapeutic relationships were established with community care providers; and (b) a friendship model of peer support (Forchuk, Jewell, et al., 1998; Forchuk, Schofield, et al., 1998; Schofield et al., 1997).

The pilot was successful in improving the discharge rate; there were 11 clients discharged the initial year with only two brief readmissions. Quality of life improved significantly for those discharged as well as those who remained on the ward (Forchuk, Chan, et al., 1998). The differences in costs of this approach compared with those of continued hospitalization were just under $0.5 million CDN (Forchuk, Chan, et al., 1998). The pilot became the ongoing model of care and all 38 clients originally on the ward were discharged by 1999, and since 1997, the average length of stay has been around ten months, with an average of 38 discharges per year.

The ward census has been reduced to 30 clients. Many clients went on to independent living in apartments and competitive gainful employment (Schofield et al., 1997).

Although the pilot study findings were positive, there was no comparison group and no randomization. The client population was not typical since the length of hospital stay had been so prolonged. A recent pilot study on acute admission wards in Scotland replicated the results of the "Bridge to Discharge" pilot study. Clients from three acute admission wards were randomized on the day of discharge to either TDM or usual follow-up care. The TDM was offered by a group of transitional nurses and trained peer volunteers. Fewer symptoms, fewer readmissions, and better functioning were noted among clients randomized to the TDM group (Reynolds et al., 2004). Although these initial studies were promising, a test with a wider range of psychiatric wards was needed to determine if the model would be useful across a range of psychiatric wards.

Objectives and Hypotheses

The overall objective of this study was to assist individuals hospitalized with a persistent mental illness in successful community living. Specific objectives were to determine the cost and effectiveness of a TDM of care and compare the results to those of a standard model of discharge care. Outcome measures included quality of life and costs. It was hypothesized that in the year following discharge from a psychiatric hospital, individuals participating in the TDM would: (a) have an improved quality of life and (b) incur fewer health and social services costs compared with individuals receiving standard discharge care. The specific health and social costs to be addressed in this analysis were hospital admissions, emergency room use, and jail/incarceration.

Methods

The study employed a cluster-randomized design (Donner & Klar, 1994). Clusters, or units of randomization, were 26 wards located in four provincial psychiatric hospitals in Ontario, Canada. Units of analysis were the clients discharged from wards. This design eliminated the logistical problems and risk of increased contamination posed by treating selected clients differently on the same ward. A total of 26 wards from four hospital sites located in Southern Ontario were paired and then randomized to either the experimental group using the new TDM or to the control group receiving usual care. The number of participating wards at each site ranged from five to eight.

Pairing of wards was based on similarity of length of stay, staffing levels, current discharge practice, and the general focus of the ward (e.g., admission; forensic; specialized diagnostic groups such as schizophrenia, mood disorders, or developmental disability). An additional six wards agreed to participate but were unable to do so as there were no appropriate matches. The paired matching ensured similarity between the intervention and control groups. It was anticipated that the pair matching would be broken for analysis purposes, given the likelihood that matching would only be slightly to moderately effective (Diehr et al., 1995).

Sample Size Calculation

To detect differences between groups, *t*-tests with a power of 0.80 and a significance level of 0.05 (one-tailed) were used based on Cohen (1988) and previous score results from the Lehman Quality of Life Instrument-Brief Version (QOLI-Brief; Lehman et al., 1995) and the anticipation of a medium effect size required a minimum sample size of 64 per group when randomization of individuals is used. Similar calculations using other outcome measures yielded smaller sample requirements. To account for the cluster randomization, the method recommended by Donner et al. (1981) was used to adjust the initial calculation; this brought the minimum sample to 125 per group. This was further inflated by 30% to adjust for drop-outs and 20% for possible contamination between intervention and control groups. Thus, the minimum sample was set at 188 per group (or 376 total).

Implementation of TDM

The TDM consisted of the same two components as found successful in the pilot: (a) overlap of inpatient and community staff in which the inpatient staff continued their relationship with clients until the clients had a working relationship with a community care provider; and (b) peer support was available to the client for a minimum of one year.

Overlap of Staff

In order to implement the new model, each staff person on the intervention wards was given 12 hours of training. The staff were to continue their relationship with the client until the community care provider was in the working phase of a therapeutic relationship. The working phase of the relationship started when the client was comfortable identifying problems to be worked on within the context of their therapeutic relationship. A consensus between hospital staff, community staff, and the consumer was used to determine this. The decision was assisted by the use of the Relationship Form (Forchuk & Brown, 1989). The time for this varied from zero weeks to 12 months, but the median time of bridging relations between the ward staff and client was three months. Weekly ward-staff contact included home visits, telephone contact, and/or meeting at an agreed location. The community care provider might also be present at these meetings. The focus of these meetings was to support the development of the therapeutic relationship with the community care provider. If the client was returning to a former community care provider, it was determined whether or not there was already a therapeutic relationship with that community care provider by reviewing the relationship form with the client. If a working therapeutic relationship existed, the ward staff did not need to continue seeing the client after discharge.

Peer Support

Former consumers of the mental health care system who had been in the community for at least a year and had completed a peer-training program provided by one of 17 participating consumer-survivor groups provided the peer support. Peer volunteers promoted friendship, provided understanding, taught community living skills, and encouraged current clients in making the transition from psychiatric hospital to the community. Common activities included having a coffee together, visiting free community events, or having a telephone conversation. Peer support volunteers were screened, trained, and provided with ongoing support from part-time volunteer coordinators within the consumer/survivor organizations. Eleven of the groups received funds from The Trillium Foundation (Government of Ontario), which was primarily used to fund peer support volunteer coordinators. The average cost for each peer support coordinator was $24,000 CDN for a 0.6 full-time equivalent. Although the coordinators were paid, the peer supporters were volunteers. Over 300 volunteers were trained.

Ethics Review

Ethical approval was obtained from the research ethics boards at the University of Western Ontario as well as the hospital sites. Participation in both the study and the intervention (if in intervention group) was voluntary.

Sample and Data Collection

A total of 390 clients were enrolled in the study. Interviews took place at the point of discharge, 1-month post-discharge, 6-months post-discharge, and 1-year post-discharge. At 1-year post-discharge, 249 individuals remained in the sample (a 36% drop-out rate). The sample size calculation had assumed a drop-out rate of 30%, which was slightly less than what occurred. The high drop-out rate was related to difficulty in tracking people who moved after discharge.

Instruments

Data were collected from individual participants using a demographic questionnaire, the Lehman QOLI-Brief (Lehman, 1988; Lehman et al., 1995), a modified form of the Utilization of Health & Social Services (UHSS; Browne et al., 1990), the Discharge/Process of Follow-up Questionnaire (DPFQ), and the Criteria for Degree of Treatment Implementation Form (CDTIF). Investigators developed the demographic instrument and the last two instruments specifically for this study. In addition, wards and consumer groups sent monthly reports summarizing any unusual events, issues, or concerns.

Analysis

Descriptive analysis was completed on all variables; *t*-tests were used to test the hypotheses comparing intervention and control groups. The level of statistical significance was set at .05 and the tests were unidirectional as the hypotheses were unidirectional. According to Chow (1996), the decision to conduct unidirectional tests requires the hypotheses to be unidirectional a priori, as was done in this study. If the stated hypotheses had been non-directional, convention would require all tests to be two-tailed.

Results

Characteristics of Participants

The characteristics of the participants who were enrolled in the study are summarized in Table 11.1. The intervention and control participants appeared similar at enrolment and therefore additional variables were not controlled for during the analysis. As the study did not include any medical record review, the diagnoses were self-reported and may not be fully accurate. A significant difference between the two groups was length of stay after the intervention had been put in place and patient enrolment began. The average length of stay for the control ward participants was 333.5 days, while the average length of stay for the intervention ward participants was 217.5 days. The baseline data of wards' (prior to randomization) average length of stay had been less than one day's difference between intervention and control wards.

Degree of Implementation/Contamination

The degree of implementation/contamination was evaluated at individual interviews with each data collection interview. All discharged clients were asked questions to determine if they were

Table 11.1 Participant Demographic and Baseline Characteristics by Group

Characteristics	Control (n=189)	Intervention (n=201)
Female	87 (46%)	103 (51.2%)
Male	102 (54%)	98 (48.8%)
Age-mean years (SD)	39.5 10.7	43.4 (11.3)
Age of onset of illness	18–83	18–70
Total lifetime psychiatric hospitalization (years)	20.8	21.9
Length of admission (days)	2.5	2.1
Mean (SD)	333.5 (1068.5)	217.5 (498.5)
Primary diagnosis (self-reported)	n=185[1]	n=199[1]
Schizophrenia	98 (53.0%)	82 (41.2%)
Mood disorder	64 (36.4%)	91 (45.7%)
Substance related	0 (0.0%)	1 (0.5%)
Personality disorder	4 (2.2%)	8 (4.0%)
Anxiety disorder	2 (1.1%)	3 (1.5%)
Developmental delay	4 (2.2%)	6 (3.0%)
Organic disorder	3 (1.6%)	0 (0.0%)
Schizoaffective disorder	1 (0.5%)	2 (1.0%)
Other	9 (4.9%)	6 (3.0%)

[1]Includes those who knew a diagnosis only.
Forchuk, C., Martin, M.-L., Chan, Y.-C., & Jensen, E. (2005). Therapeutic relationships: From psychiatric hospital to community. *Journal of Psychiatric and Mental Health Nursing, 12*, 556–564. https://doi.org/10.1111/j.1365-2850.2005.00873.x

receiving peer support and ongoing contact with hospital staff. At all times the intervention group received more of the intervention than the control group. The degree of implementation achieved was 38% overall in the intervention group and 26.6% in the control group.

Implementing the peer support was done only 22% of the time on the intervention wards and 17% on the control wards. Overlapping the services from hospital to community was implemented 54% of the time on the intervention wards and 37.7% of the time on the control wards. As the study progressed past the initial nine months, control wards started to increasingly implement the intervention. Issues related to information about implementation were gathered qualitatively through ward and consumer group data and will be described in a different report.

Hypotheses

Hypothesis one stated that within one year, the participants who received the intervention would have a better quality of life. The intervention group did not have a significant improvement in global quality of life (control group mean of 4.65, SD = 1.31; intervention mean = 4.78, SD = 1.31, $F(1, 22) = 0.38$, $p = .27$). Similarly, the sub-scales were not significantly improved. The exception was that quality of life related to social relations where the specific area targeted by the intervention was improved significantly [$F(1, 22) = 6.99$, $p = .015$].

Hypothesis two stated that individuals participating in the TDM would incur fewer health and social service costs after discharge compared to individuals receiving standard care. Key indicators of consumption of health and social services were examined. The use of hospital and emergency room services were selected for analysis since they are the costliest services likely to be accessed. In the first year after discharge, the intervention group consumed $4400 CDN less in hospital and emergency room services, per person, than the control group. However, this was not statistically significant ($p = .09$). Jail and legal event costs were to be compared but they occurred too infrequently for any meaningful analysis. Specifically, only one participant had one day in jail for the year after discharge.

Discussion

The hypotheses related to post-discharge hospital costs and quality of life were not supported by this trial. However, the length of stay was significantly less for participants enrolled on the intervention wards, despite no difference between length of stay on intervention and control wards prior to the implementation of the intervention. The reduced length of stay on the intervention wards was not predicted a priori but may well have contributed to the difficulty in detecting differences after discharge. Although the pilot study had resulted in shorter lengths of stay, hospital partners in this trial were emphatic that due to recent cutbacks and bed closures, further reductions in length of stay were not realistic. Monthly reports from all wards revealed the only ward level change between intervention and control wards had been the introduction of the TDM being tested by the study. Hospital staff first alerted the researchers to the shortening length of stay through monthly ward reports and feedback from the staff training. Feedback from two intervention wards at two different hospitals made the observation that with the TDM change in practice, "People are leaving in six weeks instead of six months." Staff reported that with the support that the TDM provided, they felt comfortable discharging clients earlier. At a rate of $632.30 CDN per day for the cost of a bed in a psychiatric hospital, the people in the intervention group consumed $12,212,242 CDN less in hospital services than the control group prior to discharge. Despite this shorter length of stay (average 116 fewer days per person), the intervention group did not access more hospital services after discharge. It is recommended that future study of similar interventions include an examination of length of stay.

Both under-implementation by some intervention wards and contamination (i.e., the control wards using the intervention) were issues. The training strategies used may have been inadequate to promote this change. In a separate evaluation of the training, staff indicated that although 66.7% felt more able to successfully bridge clients to the community after the training, only 34.8% reported actually doing this (Martin et al., 2002). It was noted that some staff were never chosen to bridge with clients although they had received the training. Some reasons given for this included part time hours, lack of therapeutic relationship, sickness, and working very few day shifts. This could also reflect the difficulty in changing individual and hospital system practice. Also, some clients on the control wards sought out peer support after discharge. Towards the end of the enrollment process, two control wards contacted two different consumer groups in an effort to establish a relationship and systematic method of referral, despite an agreement that they would not do so. In both cases, the consumer groups requested the wards wait until the end of the study. However, individual clients seeking peer help from the consumer groups, even if from control wards, were not turned down. Shortly after the study sample was enrolled (but not completely followed-up), one hospital implemented a peer support program based on a belief that this was making a difference to the client discharge experience and re-admission. All of these issues related to contamination and under-implementation reduced the effect size. There was far less difference in practice between implementation and control wards than anticipated. These issues illustrate the 'messiness' of systems research compared with, for example, a classic drug trial. Vingilis and Pederson (2001) describe some of the multiple reasons that findings of intervention failure may be misleading. These reasons include inadequate implementation, inadequate strength of intervention, and measurement that is not sufficiently sensitive. The first two reasons were clearly factors in this study.

Conclusion

With the reduction of psychiatric hospital beds, there is a demand for quality mental health services to be provided within the community. This study compared a TDM to usual discharge practices with clients who have a chronic mental illness. The TDM included peer support and bridging relationships with hospital staff until a working therapeutic relationship was established with the community care provider. This model assisted individuals hospitalized with a chronic mental illness to achieve successful community living. Hypotheses related to improved quality of life and fewer post-discharge costs for the intervention group were unsupported. The participants on the intervention wards were discharged 116 days earlier than the control wards. Although this was not predicted a priori, it is clinically significant. Both under-implementation on intervention wards and contamination on control wards occurred and reduced the potential effect size. This study is an example of some of the challenges encountered in health systems research, where the use of the intervention cannot be rigorously controlled.

Acknowledgments

This research was supported by grants from the Canadian Health Services Research Foundation, the Lawson Health Research Institute, the Donner Canadian Foundation, and by in-kind support from: Mountain Centre for Health Services, St. Joseph's Healthcare Hamilton (formerly Hamilton Psychiatric Hospital), Regional Mental Health Care, St. Joseph's Healthcare, London/ St. Thomas (formerly London/St. Thomas Psychiatric Hospital), Whitby Mental Health Centre. Support for the peer support program was received from the Ontario Trillium Foundation. We would like to thank the psychiatric consumer-survivors who participated throughout the project.

12 Peer Support

Cheryl Forchuk, Michelle Solomon, and Tazim Virani

The Mental Health Commission of Canada defines peer support as "a supportive relationship between people who have a lived experience in common...in relation to a mental health challenge or illness...related to their own mental health or that of a loved one" (Sunderland et al., 2013, p.11). In Ontario, a key resource for peer support is the Ontario Peer Development Initiative (OPDI), which is an umbrella organization of mental health Consumer/Survivor Initiatives (CSIs) and Peer Support Organizations across the Province of Ontario. Member organizations are run by and for people with lived experience of a mental health or addiction issue and provide a wide range of services and activities within their communities. The central tenet of member organizations is the common understanding that people can and do recover with the proper supports in place and that peer support is integral to successful recovery. This paper focuses on a range of diverse peer support groups and CSIs that operate in London and surrounding areas.

Peer Support in Region

A review of peer support programs in the South West Local Health Integration Network (South West LHIN) region identified eight programs that were publicly funded through the South West LHIN and operated by a CSI. The programs were assessed against promising practice criteria for peer support identified in the literature. The majority of South West LHIN peer support models used by CSIs were based on an informal peer support model or a walk-in center. In addition, some of the programs also used a formal/intentional peer support model. However, since intentional peer support was often reported in the absence of formal matching (i.e., formal matching being a key element of formal peer support), it may be possible that the identification of a formal/intentional peer support model was used more broadly than intended. The table (see Table 12.1) from Sunderland et al. (2013) denotes a spectrum of peer support models that range from friendship to clinical care. Peer support models used in the South West LHIN were more aligned to the friendship end of the spectrum of models (see Table 12.2) (Mings & Cramp, 2014). In addition, most of the beneficiaries of peer support were identified through word of mouth, outreach, and community referrals. In some instances, referrals were made by mental health professionals where some linkages were established – the majority of which were not formalized. The transitional discharge model (TDM) research study implemented in the London area provided interactions between some of the CSIs and mental healthcare professionals and service organizations.

The major gaps in the South West LHIN were the relative absence of peer support programs in workplace and clinical settings (e.g., community or hospital); although, with the advent of the introduction of the TDM studies, several partnerships had resulted between CSIs and

Table 12.1 Spectrum of Peer Support Models

Friendship	**Informal Peer Support** – naturally occurring, voluntary, reciprocal relationships with peers one-on-one or possibly in a community
	Clubhouse/Walk-in Center – mainly psychosocial and social recreational focus with peer support naturally occurring among participants
	Self-Help, Mutual Peer Support – consumer-operated/run organization and activities, voluntary, naturally occurring, reciprocal relationships with peers in community settings
	Formalized/Intentional Peer Support – consumer-run peer support services within community settings: group or one-on-one, focusing on issues such as education, employment, MH systems navigation, systemic/individual advocacy, housing, food security, Internet, transportation, recovery education, anti-discrimination work, etc.
	Workplace Peer Support – workplace-based programs where employees with lived experience are selected and prepared to provide peer support to other employees within their workplace
	Community Clinical Setting Peer Support – peer supporters selected to provide support to patients/clients that utilize clinical services, e.g., outpatient, ACT teams, case management, counselling
Clinical Care	**Clinical/Conventional MH System-Based Peer Support** – clinical setting, inpatient/outpatient, institutional peer support, multidisciplinary groups, recovery centers, or rehabilitation centers crisis response, crisis management, emergency rooms, acute wards

Forchuk, C., Solomon, M., & Virani, T. (2016). Peer support: An important part of transitional discharge. *Healthcare Quarterly, 18*(special issue), 32–36. https://doi.org/10.12927/hcq.2016.24480

professional services in hospitals. Once the two-year study grant (funded through the Council of Academic Hospitals of Ontario) came to an end, there were concerns that this type of model would not be sustained, even though there were positive health and system outcomes.

CONNECT for Mental Health

One example of a group providing peer support is CONNECT for Mental Health Inc. (CONNECT). CONNECT is a non-profit peer support organization run by and for individuals who have been affected by mental illness. It was founded in 2007 by Michelle Solomon, who was driven by her own experiences with mental health issues and her own need for peer support. As a student nurse, Michelle started a group at the Fanshawe College Student Union, sharing her story and letting others know they were not alone. Her strong vision to create a peer support organization in London was met with the belief by other consumer/survivors, and in 2011, CONNECT became an official non-profit organization.

CONNECT's vision is to promote sustainable systems of support that enable individuals affected by mental illness to thrive and maintain wellness in the community. To do this, CONNECT embarks on a three-fold mission:

1. *Supporting* individuals affected by mental illness.
2. *Educating* a wide audience on relevant mental health topics.
3. Providing *outreach* to the community to help decrease stigma and promote early intervention of mental health disorders.

CONNECT focuses on engaging youth and young adult populations and maintaining face-to-face contact with individuals in the community. Meetings occur at the local library, coffee

Table 12.2 Peer Support Programs in the SW LHIN and Types of Models Employed

Peer Support Program	Informal Model	Walk-In Center/ Activity Center	Clubhouse Model	Self-Help, Mutual	Formalized/ Intentional Peer Support	Workplace Model	Family Model	Community Clinical Setting Model	Clinical/ Conventional MH System-Based Model
1	Yes	No	No	No	Yes	No	Yes	No	No
2	Yes	Yes	Somewhat	Somewhat	Somewhat	Yes	No	No	No
3	Yes	Yes	Yes	Yes	No	Yes	No	No	No
4	Yes	Yes	No	Somewhat	Somewhat	No	No	No	No
5	Yes	Yes	Yes	Yes	Yes	No	Yes	Yes	Yes
6	Yes	Yes	Yes	Yes	Yes	No	No	Somewhat	No
7	Yes	No	No	No	Yes	No	No	No	No
8	No	No	No	No	Yes	No	No	No	No

Forchuk, C., Solomon, M., & Virani, T. (2016). Peer support: An important part of transitional discharge. *Healthcare Quarterly, 18*(special issue), 32–36. https://doi.org/10.12927/hcq.2016.24480

shop, and in community spaces. There is an emphasis on "getting into action for mental health," where individuals are encouraged to be an active participant and expert in their own recovery. Volunteers offer emotional support, support that encourages positive coping and self-management of mental illness. To date, CONNECT has over 50 volunteers who offer both group and one-to-one peer support services. Volunteers are recruited through venues, such as Kijiji and social media, and are then trained in peer support through CONNECT and the Ontario Peer Development Initiative's (OPDI) Peer Support Core Essentials Program.

Support

CONNECT provides peer support in group settings. The longest running program is the weekly coffee "socials" where individuals drop in to gain emotional support from others who have "been there." There is also an eight week "Recovery Group" that started in 2012 that addresses topics that promote self-management and the exploration of tools to help prevent crises and maintain wellness. This group occurs at the local Canadian Mental Health Association. In 2013, CONNECT started a "Student Support Group" at Western University for students in need of support with mental health and school.

CONNECT partnered with Lawson Health Research Institute, London Health Sciences Centre, and OPDI in 2013 to provide transitional support to individuals being discharged from the hospital. "The Transitional Discharge Model," funded by the Council of Academic Hospitals of Ontario (CAHO), expanded CONNECT's provision of peer support in the community. In this program, peer coordinators have a presence on the hospital ward, offering peer support to clients and also matching clients with volunteers who further support peers in the community after their discharge. Furthermore, in 2014, St. Joseph's Health Care Parkwood Institute invited CONNECT to offer peer support to their clients, allowing CONNECT to provide support to individuals who are in hospital for longer periods of time.

Education

As a consumer/survivor voice, CONNECT works with organizations in the community to provide education to the public on topics concerning mental illness and recovery. From 2008 to 2012, CONNECT partnered with the London Public Library (central branch) to provide workshops on various mental disorders and mental health and to raise awareness about supports. To date, CONNECT partners with organizations who want to provide information and raise public awareness on mental health.

Outreach

In addition to working with community organizations to facilitate educational events, CONNECT has an "Outreach Team" whose purpose is to connect with the community, particularly with youth, to decrease stigma associated with mental illness, promote early intervention, and connect individuals to peer support. Volunteers share their personal experience with mental illness and recovery through public speeches. Venues include Western University and other public forums in the community.

Local Innovation and Consumer Survivor Groups Involvement in Research

CSIs have a long involvement in research generally. This is illustrated with the involvement in the transitional discharge model (TDM). The TDM is an evidence-based approach that includes

Vision: Create a vision for the group. What is the group trying to achieve?
Audience: Who is the audience?
Goals: What are the needs of the group and how will you meet those needs?
Guidelines/Contract: How will people share? Is everyone expected to share? What topics will not be discussed?
Facilitation: Are the facilitators trained in peer support? Is this training evidence based?
Topics/Discussion: Will there be specific topics? Are topics evidence based? Is discussion random or structured?
Crisis Management: How will adverse events be handled to maintain the safety of the group?
Boundaries: Participants are experts on their experience and don't give advice. Use "I" language. It's social support, not clinical support.
Resources: Be able to connect participants to resources that can further help them.

Figure 12.1 Tips for Starting a Peer Support Group from CONNECT. Forchuk, C., Solomon, M., & Virani, T. (2016). Peer support: An important part of transitional discharge. *Healthcare Quarterly*, *18*(special issue), 32–36. https://doi.org/10.12927/hcq.2016.24480.

both peer support and continued involvement of inpatient staff until a therapeutic relationship has been established with the community care provider (Forchuk et al., 2007a, 2007b; Forchuk et al., 2013). It was originally developed through a participatory action research project including frontline hospital and community staff, consumers who were currently hospitalized, as well as ones who had successfully made the transition to community, and researchers. More recently, TDM was identified as a best practice by the Council of Academic Hospitals of Ontario (CAHO, n.d.). CAHO supported an implementation project to extend the model. Two London hospitals, the London Health Sciences Centre and St. Joseph's Health Care London, OPDI, and local peer support organizations were recently involved with London as the lead site.

The TDM was implemented in collaboration with OPDI on 14 wards (eight tertiary, six acute) in nine hospitals across Ontario. Peer Support Coordinators and volunteers/workers based out of CSIs partnered with participating hospital wards to offer the peer support component of the TDM. The average length of stay on the participating wards dropped by an average of 9.8 days, which freed up the equivalent of approximately $33 million CDN. Also, consumers being discharged reported feeling better supported and less anxious in making the transition to the community.

Recent Region-Wide Work

A key South West LHIN peer support strategy is the development of partnerships between CSIs and mental healthcare programs in the community and in hospital. A stakeholder engagement process was used to identify the following hopes, aspirations, and outcomes that stakeholders wished to achieve:

- **Region-wide acceptance** of peer support as a valid and effective intervention.
- **Availability of peer support** wherever individuals are in their recovery journey – community, hospital, outpatient, work, and school, as well as wherever they live in the region – urban, rural, or remote locations.
- **Appropriate and sustainable funding** to support implementation of models based on promising practices.
- **CSIs and Mental Health providers** working in a **true partnership** – as true partners, peer supporters are part of the planning and ongoing oversight of mental health and addiction programs.
- **Standards** for peer support practices are linked with accountability.

- Continuous support and improvement of **existing peer support programs** while filling the gaps with **new models** where these are needed, such as models that **include partnership with clinical agencies**. Expand mandates of existing programs, where appropriate and feasible, to address gaps.
- Peer support programs – no matter where they exist – in CSI or in mental healthcare teams – are part of a **peer support network of sharing and learning**.

Conclusion

Using evidence-based approaches, CSIs and peer support organizations in London, Ontario, as well as throughout the local health integration network, are working together in partnership with others to provide strong support to individuals with mental health and addiction issues. The groups in the area have a strong history and are continuing to evolve to address the needs of people with the experience of mental health and addiction challenges.

13 Implementation of a Transitional Discharge Model

Clients', Health Professionals', and Peer Supporters' Perspectives

Boniface Harerimana, Sebastian Gyamfi, and Cheryl Forchuk

Over the last three decades, there has been worldwide efforts towards integrating people with mental illness into the community and improving their access to mental healthcare within the community (Forchuk et al., 2020; Forchuk, Jewell, et al., 1998; Forchuk, Martin, Sherman, et al., 2019). Current discharge practices leave clients in a 'transitional gap' after leaving the hospital if community supports are not arranged. This gap in care threatens the continuity of treatment and delays the types of supports available during the transition (Olfson et al., 2000; Vigo et al., 2016), resulting in clients depending more on expensive emergency services (Dekker et al., 2013). There is a need for tailored mental health interventions that enhance clients' experiences with mental healthcare and ensure a safety net of support for community reintegration post-discharge. An intervention that focuses on an integrated transition for clients is necessary for successful de-hospitalization (Sussman, 1998) and meeting the needs of clients for community integration (Drury, 2008).

Careful discharge planning is at the centre point of transitioning clients from the hospital to the community (Forchuk , Jewell, et al., 1998), but the involvement of peer supporters in community-based mental healthcare creates a more natural transition that has demonstrated a seamless impact on clients' health outcomes. Peer-run support programs improve psychiatric recovery through clients' commitment to and engagement in the community integration process (Dalgin et al., 2018; Kaplan et al., 2012; Salyers et al., 2009). Peer supporters facilitate clients in establishing caring and friendship-based networks, which in turn improve their recovery and community integration (Hardiman, 2004; Ochocka et al., 2006). Hardiman (2004) indicated that caring networks obtained through peer support create a safe environment wherein clients feel accepted, secure, and empowered for making human connections within their communities. Research that examined the outcomes of clients' participation in peer initiatives have linked peer support to clients' sense of wellbeing in a safe environment (Ochocka et al., 2006). In a study involving a sample of people with severe mental illness in Canada, participants who were active in peer-led initiatives experienced a sense of being welcomed, which encouraged them to engage actively in social interactions, facilitating their community integration (Ochocka et al., 2006). Additionally, peer-led interventions have the potential for reducing hospitalizations and sustaining recovery among individuals suffering from mental illness (Min et al., 2007). In light of the advantages of peer support, successful community integration is subject to several factors. This chapter discusses evidence on the client transition from the hospital to the community using findings from a study that implemented the transitional discharge model (TDM). It reports on the perspectives of clients with mental illness, healthcare professionals, and peer supporters on their involvement in the study.

Methods

This ethnographic qualitative study used a mixed-methods approach to evaluate the implementation of the TDM across nine hospitals in Ontario, Canada. The study involved 87 clients, 216 healthcare professionals, and 66 peer supporters. Details about recruitment and eligibility criteria for participating in the study have been reported elsewhere (Forchuk et al., 2020; Forchuk, Martin, Sherman, et al., 2019).

Data Collection

Two sets of focus groups were organized for clients, healthcare professionals, and peer supporters at each participating hospital, specifically at six and 12 months after the TDM implementation. All participating groups attended both sets of focus groups, and each focus group lasted one to two hours. Data collected during the focus groups were digitally recorded and transcribed verbatim. During the focus groups, notetakers gathered field notes, observations about group dynamics, context, and non-verbal information (LeCompte & Schensul, 1999). This descriptive information was integrated into the transcribed data for analysis (Forchuk et al., 2020; Forchuk, Martin, Sherman, et al., 2019).

Data Analysis Approach

Data were analyzed using Leininger's (1985) ethnography model of qualitative data analysis. Specifically, data analysis consisted of extensively reading focus group transcripts in order to identify distinct descriptors. The descriptors were used to identify recurring themes, which were organized into major themes. Data analysis involved refining, defining, and describing formulated themes by exemplar quotes from transcripts. Themes were analyzed for their meaning about the context of participants from which data was collected. The credibility of findings was enhanced by having all co-researchers discuss their individual observations and then comment on the preliminary results, which were then combined and integrated into the final results (Graneheim & Lundman, 2004).

Results

Data from the focus groups illustrated three major themes that expressed the perceptions of clients, healthcare professionals, and peer supporters who participated in the TDM study. The major themes included: Perceived benefits of implementing the TDM, challenges hindering the TDM implementation, and suggested strategies for improving the TDM implementation. Under each of these major themes, the co-investigators identified both common and group-specific views concerning participants' experiences of the TDM study. Table 13.1 summarizes the major themes and corresponding common and group-specific subthemes of participants' views. For the sake of this chapter, only common themes that reflect shared perspectives among the three groups of participants are discussed.

Perceived Benefits of Implementing the TDM

Common themes about the effectiveness of implementing the TDM was expressed through the benefits observed by participating groups. Shared views about the benefits of the TDM among all groups included offering hope, establishing a safety net, enhanced recovery, and TDM as a source of appropriate social connectedness.

Table 13.1 A Matrix of Common and Group-Specific Subthemes of Participants' Perceptions

Major Themes	Common Subthemes	Group-Specific Subthemes		
		Clients	Healthcare Professionals	Peer Supporters
Perceived benefits of the TDM intervention	Offering hope Establishing a safety net Enhanced recovery TDM as a source of appropriate social connectedness	Reduced feelings of isolation Peer support as a suitable friendship	TDM served as a framework for discharge planning Bridging the gap between the hospital and the community	Promoting clients' autonomy Working with clients to develop and to set goals
Encountered challenges	Issues with communication	Issues with trust Initial fears about discharge	Concerns from some physicians re maintaining responsibility post-discharge when no community agency yet involved Lack of enough peer supporters	Issues with matching volunteers to clients Concerns about personal safety and vulnerability
Suggested strategies for improving the TDM	Improving communication Standardizing TDM practice	Raising awareness of resources available in the community	Clarifying roles for members of the team	Dealing with matching issues

Peer Support Offers Hope to Clients

Social interactions between the participating groups encouraged the sharing of experiences that helped clients to develop positive perspectives and outlooks about life during the transition from the hospital to their communities. Through the exchange between clients and peer supporters and clients and healthcare professionals, clients felt reassured and hopeful of a smooth transition from the hospital to their community. One peer supporter described the experience of their involvement in the TDM as follows: "When they hear that we've gone through these things too, and they see that…we're surviving, and we're out in the community, and we're here to help…it's okay to talk to us, and it gives them hope."

Establishing a Safety Net

The participating groups observed that the TDM served as a safety net for clients. For instance, peer supporters expressed that a safety net was established by maintaining contact with clients and ensuring that they did not "fall through the cracks" after discharge. One peer supporter noted:

> …a lot of people fall off the radar in terms of their mental health needs after they leave the hospital, and I hope their needs will be addressed ongoing…because I think so many people, after they are discharged from the hospital, they just fall through the cracks.

Enhanced Recovery

Data from focus groups revealed that the TDM improved clients' health outcomes by reducing rates of hospital readmissions. Client participants felt that bridging relationships prevented hospital readmissions by improving connectedness between staff, peer supporters, clients, and families. This connectedness also enabled families or clients to contact healthcare professionals when early signs of relapse occurred. To emphasize these TDM benefits, one healthcare professional said the following: "The family knew [whom] to call because they were connected with us. They are part of TDM, they managed to come to the emergency department and avoid an admission."

TDM as a Source of Appropriate Social Connectedness

People with mental illness can potentially experience distressing loss of social contacts. Clients who received the TDM could compensate for this potential loss by forming relationships with peer supporters who were able to empathize with the experience of mental illness. The following illustrates a client's feelings:

> I don't think I could be where I am without peer support. My peer support really listens... probably is one of the best people for this program. My peer really has the heart, and cares about me. The program [TDM] is amazing.

Encountered Challenges

Challenges encountered among all participating groups involved issues with communication, which resulted, in part, from the lack of interprofessional collaboration in decision-making regarding the client's care and from healthcare professionals and peer supporters not exchanging detailed information relevant to the TDM. This finding was illustrated by a healthcare professional as follows:

> ...it's been a bit difficult, sometimes making the connection to the peer supporters, because sometimes we don't always know the discharge dates, sometimes, doctors just decide... to discharge patients with not a lot of notice...they [peer supporters] say "like why didn't you give us more notice?"

Suggested Strategies for Improving the TDM

Improving Communication

Participants expressed concerns about communication, such as not being informed of clients' progress when things were not working well. Subsequently, healthcare professionals suggested active interprofessional communication as a strategy, wherein each member of the healthcare team is informed of decisions regarding clients and any positive progress noted after discharge. Participating groups emphasized the need to discuss priorities and arrangements for discharge, as well as plans for connecting with peer supporters. Exemplar statements below expressed healthcare professionals' suggestions for improving communication:

> It's nice to get updates as to how discharged clients are doing.

> I guess direct communication between people at the front line with people higher up that are kind of overseeing the project [will help].

Standardizing TDM Practice

Participating groups suggested ways of standardizing the TDM practice. For instance, peer supporters expressed a need for more training about how to interact with clients, avoiding sources of triggers, and skills for effectively managing problems that may arise in the course of their interactions with clients. Additionally, healthcare professionals asserted that the TDM information resources, such as brochures, flyers, posters, and postcards (see some examples in the TDM Toolkit in this book), could inform clients and their families about the TDM and enable them to make an informed choice about participating more easily. Below is an exemplar quote from a healthcare provider:

> If there is something like standardized that you use for all the different units so that would be [better]…I think with the idea of having the posters and postcards would be a good thing, that patients know about it…

Discussion

The purpose of the TDM study was to examine the perspectives of clients, healthcare professionals, and peer supporters regarding their involvement in an intervention that uses relationships to support clients who are recovering from mental illness as they integrate in the community. The study found that participants held a wide range of perspectives regarding the benefits and challenges associated with their involvement in the TDM, as well as strategies for the way forward. This chapter is limited to the shared perspective among the three groups of participants (i.e., clients, peer supporters, and healthcare providers).

This study highlighted common benefits among all participants. With regard to the effectiveness of implementing the TDM, participants expressed various advantages that included offering hope, establishing a safety net, enhanced recovery, and the TDM acting as a source of social networking and connectedness. Participants revealed that the in-person interactions among them created a safety net for clients and reinforced hope in recovery. For instance, peer supporters involved in the TDM intervention created a safety net by being a consistent contact, which clients could rely on for both emotional support and general information. These findings corroborate what researchers (Hardiman, 2004; Ochocka et al., 2006) referred to as caring networks, which are established through creating a safe environment and promoting clients' acceptance and empowerment during their interactions with peer supporters. The study's findings illustrated that allocating peer supporters to clients who were leaving the hospital facilitated a smooth transition to the community and resulted in fewer hospital readmissions for clients (Forchuk et al., 2020). A key factor in reducing hospital readmissions, which subsequently saved costs on healthcare, was the fact that peer supporters maintained a consistent presence during clients' transition into the community (Min et al., 2007).

Peer supporters assumed many roles in the community integration of clients who were receiving the TDM intervention. They assisted clients to build capacity and develop a routine, attended regular on-ward and community meetings, accompanied clients to their appointments, advocated with other professionals, and worked with clients to develop goals and set new targets. Results relating to peer supporters' roles showed consistency with findings from previous studies (Haynes & Strode, 2011; Moll et al., 2009; Rivera et al., 2007), except in helping clients to build their capacity and develop a routine, which seemed to be unique to the TDM intervention (Forchuk et al., 2020). These results underscore the role of peer supporters in bridging services and closing the gap in mental healthcare as clients transitioned from the hospital to the community. They also suggest that peer support involvement constitutes a sensible and valuable component of mental healthcare, with a potential positive impact on the recovery of both previous and current clients who are enduring a transition. A review of 38 studies by Graneheim and Lundman (2004) demonstrated that peer support in mental health services improved health outcomes, such as reducing hospital readmission rates and enhancing recovery. In summary, these findings demonstrate that peer supporters can be involved in multiple roles that aim to enhance clients' autonomy – a driving force for their engagement in healthcare, which prior studies have linked to better health outcomes and successful community integration (Dalgin et al., 2018; Drebing et al., 2018). Peer supporters helped to orient clients so they could fulfil their activities of daily living and also shared strategies for successful experiences and coping mechanisms.

Despite the above-noted contributions of study participants in improving clients' recovery and community integration, this study showed that there are still challenges to successfully implementing the TDM. A major issue encountered by participating groups involved communication. Unless tailored strategies are devised to address issues in communication, the involvement of mental health services stakeholders may not reach their full potential. In this regard, policies for improving the TDM may capitalize on strategies, such as harmonizing communication between different mental health services stakeholders and standardizing the TDM practice. These strategies are in line with suggestions from Gates and Akabas (2007) and Mancini (2018), who advocate for integrating peer supporters through institutional policies that clearly define their roles, supervision, and training and knowledge development. Indeed, findings suggest that carefully designed training, supervision, and management of both healthcare professional and peer supporters are crucial for successful implementation of community integration programs.

Conclusion

Through a network of relationships, the TDM intervention supports clients who have mental illness to integrate in the community. Benefits include promoting clients' autonomy and hope about their recovery, along with establishing a safety net while contributing to reduction in hospital readmissions. However, interprofessional communication between clients, healthcare providers, and peer supporters still needs to be improved. Supporting interprofessional communication and standardizing the TDM practice are strategies that can serve to improve this intervention.

14 Cost-Effectiveness of the Implementation of a Transitional Discharge Model for Community Integration of Psychiatric Clients

Practice Insights and Policy Implications

Cheryl Forchuk, Mary-Lou Martin, Deborah Corring, Deborrah Sherman, Rani Srivastava, Boniface Harerimana, and Raymond Cheng

Over the last decades, mental healthcare delivery systems and policies have shifted the focus from more extensive psychiatric inpatient settings to community services, particularly in industrialized countries (Júnior et al., 2016; Knapp et al., 2006; Olson, 2006; Pedersen & Kolstad, 2009; Priebe et al., 2005). The shift of focus in mental healthcare delivery has led to a significant reduction of beds in psychiatric settings (Krupinski, 1995; Priebe et al., 2005) and basing performance appraisal of healthcare systems on the quality of care provision and efficient services (Olson, 2006; Pedersen & Kolstad, 2009). Subsequent consequences include many clients discharged from psychiatric hospitals too early, discharges that are not properly planned, and post-discharge follow-up that does not function properly (Niimura et al., 2016; Pedersen & Kolstad, 2009). These outcomes are worrisome since the discharge process and community integration after hospitalization are already challenging (Walter et al., 2019). For example, many people with mental illness experience stigma and social rejection when returning to the community (Hengartner et al., 2013; Loch et al., 2014; Stuart, 2008). Besides, standard discharge practices from psychiatric wards disrupt the continuity of treatment and support available to clients during their transition, which often leaves clients with a gap in care (Olfson et al., 2000; Vigod et al., 2013), and subsequently, increased use of emergency services (Dekker et al., 2013). In the time immediately following discharge, people who have mental illnesses are not only vulnerable, but also have a high risk of readmission (Loch, 2014; Madi et al., 2007) and face a heightened risk for completing suicide, committing violent crimes, or for re-hospitalization due to interpersonal violence (Walter, et al., 2019). It is for these reasons that preventing gaps in mental healthcare is essential.

The transitional discharge model (TDM) is a comprehensive client integration program, which was developed and initially tested in Ontario, Canada by Forchuk, Jewell, et al. (1998). From clinical practice perspectives, TDM has two components to assist clients in the transition from hospital to the community (Forchuk et al., 2007b; Forchuk, Jewell, et al., 1998). The first component is peer support from a person who has experienced a mental illness, has completed a peer training program, and is living successfully in the community. Peer support includes regularly scheduled contact to learn from the experience of someone who lived through a similar transition (Forchuk, Jewell, et al., 1998). The second component of TDM consists of the continued provision of support by hospital staff until a new therapeutic relationship has been established with a community healthcare provider and peer supporter (Forchuk, Jewell, et al., 1998).

The purpose of the present study was to evaluate the cost-effectiveness of a project, which implemented TDM in nine hospital sites across Ontario. The study utilized previous research on TDM as a starting point and compared this with the TDM implementation costs and participating hospitals' spending during the intervention.

Materials and Methods

Design

This study used a participatory action research (PAR) design to implement TDM in nine hospitals across Ontario, Canada. The core principle of PAR guided the study, that is, creating a partnership that enables study participants and stakeholders to take part in all aspects of the research (Baum et al., 2006; Islam et al., 1991). Throughout the project, this high-level of collaboration created a set of implementation strategies, rooted in practice, which assisted client participants to transition into the community. The collaboration also allowed each set of strategies to be tested and refined, positioning the results of this project to be implemented in other sites. Specifically, hospital staff and peer support coordinators/volunteers worked together to implement TDM on both acute and tertiary care wards. Implementation strategies varied across all sites; however, the principles of the model focused on relationships to bridge the discharge process. An essential partnership was with the Ontario Peer Development Initiative (OPDI), which acts as a provincial voice for 48 Consumer/Survivor Initiatives and Peer Support Programs across Ontario.

Sample

In total, 370 clients between the ages of 18 and 85 were recruited to participate in this study. The inclusion criteria for clients were (a) being currently hospitalized, (b) able to understand English to the extent necessary to participate, (c) competent to consent, and (d) being discharged from a hospital unit participating in the study.

Data Collection Procedures

The project team gathered data through three primary sources: interviews with 370 clients at discharge; focus groups with clients, hospital staff, peer support volunteers, and staff; and data from hospital administration. Data related to this paper consisted of intervention cost, changes in hospital spending based on a reduced length of stay, lower readmission rates, and fewer emergency room visits.

Analysis

The cost-effectiveness of TDM implementation was assessed by calculating the cost of implementing the intervention to any changes in hospital spending (i.e., reduction of visits to emergency room, readmissions, and length of stay). Hospital spending was calculated using data from the Institute for Clinical Evaluative Sciences, an organization that houses population-based health and social data.

Results

Sample Characteristics

Among the 370 individuals who participated in the study, the average age was 42.2 years and the sample was split evenly between males and females. Most of the sample was of Caucasian descent (76.9%) and currently single (60.1%). Almost the entire sample (92.2%) was in contact with a family member. Nearly half the sample had completed high school (43.6%), with slightly less (40.6%) having completed community college or university. The most common psychiatric diagnoses were mood disorders (52.2%), anxiety disorders (24.6%), and schizophrenia or schizoaffective disorders (22.4%). On average, individuals had been hospitalized for psychiatric reasons 1.5 times in the previous year, with the duration of the most recent hospitalization lasting 41.6 days on average. On average, individuals had been hospitalized for psychiatric reasons 4.6 times in their lifetime.

Average Length of Stay

In total, ten hospital wards had complete data on length of stay before and after the implementation of TDM. In the two months before implementing the TDM, the average length of stay across these wards was 74.2 days. Four months after implementation, the average length of stay was 56.9 days, a decrease of 17.3 days from pre-implementation. Eight months after implementation, the average length of stay was 64.4 days, a reduction of 9.8 days from pre-implementation. Data related to the length of stay was abnormally distributed. A Wilcoxon Signed-Ranks test showed no statistically significant difference between pre- and post-implementation length of stay (mean rank = 6.63 vs 5.64, $Z = -.585$, $p = 0.592$). During the implementation period, many discharges were coming from the tertiary care wards. Tertiary care wards tend to have longer lengths of stay than acute care wards. Therefore, although the length of stay appears to rebound slightly as time progresses, this may not indicate that the TDM was decreasing in its effectiveness. It may suggest that TDM impacts clients with more long-term psychiatric illness by assisting in getting these clients discharged.

Cost-Effectiveness of the Intervention

The Office of the Auditor General of Ontario (2016) reported that the average cost to care for one day in a specialty psychiatric hospital was CAN $930. Therefore, a reduction in length of stay alone can produce cost savings. A decrease of 9.8 days (seen after TDM implementation) in length of stay per discharge translates to a savings of approximately CAN $9,114 per discharge. As calculations of savings were based on the overall reduction in length of stay, statistical tests for differences were not necessary. The average number of discharges per year from all nine participating wards was collected pre-implementation of TDM. On average, there were 4,000 discharges per year for the participating wards, which translates to potential savings in hospital days of CAN $36,456,000 per year if TDM remains implemented solely on the participating wards. In 2015, the Canadian Institute for Health Information (2015) estimated the number of psychiatric discharges per year at 80,638. Calculations based on these provincial estimates show potential savings on hospital days equate to CAN $734, 934,732 if TDM were implemented province wide. Savings from TDM implementation total CAN $3,392,810 per site annually, based on the intervention costs and savings attributed to the reduced length of stay. These savings significantly outweigh the value of the intervention: A peer support coordinator/ volunteer support, training of the latter, and staff time for bridging clients to the community. Table 14.1 demonstrates the expected total savings based on the cost of the intervention and reduced length of stay.

Discussion

The present study evaluated the cost-effectiveness of the implementation of TDM in nine hospital sites across Ontario, Canada. The study results have demonstrated that the savings accumulated by implementing TDM considerably outweigh the cost of the intervention. These results are consistent with previous studies, which evaluated the effectiveness of TDM (Forchuk et al., 2005; Forchuk et al., 2007b).

Table 14.1 Comparison of Costs for TDM Implementation and Savings (per Site, Annually)

Costs for TDM	*Implementation (per Site, Annually)*	
Item	*Description*	*Amount*
Peer Support Coordinator Salary	1 FTE (37.5 hours per week for 52 weeks) $25.45/hour + benefits = $30.73/hour	$59,924
Peer Support Coordinator Training	$1,000 honorarium per trainer, $1,200 for trainee for 5 days of training	$2,200
Peer Support Mileage	$500/month for travel to clients and volunteers	$6,000
Volunteer Training	50 volunteers for 5 days of training $30 materials + $20 food/person/day = $130 per volunteer	$6,500
Volunteer Recognition	Includes gift certificates to support works with clients	$5,000
TOTAL COSTS		**$79,624**
Savings from TDM (per Site, Annually)		
Reduction in Length of Stay	Reduction in LOS = 9.8 Days/Discharge Cost of Stay in Hospital = $930/Day Average Discharges Across All Sites = 381 Savings = Reduction in LOS X Cost per Day X No. of Discharges	$3,472,434
TOTAL SAVINGS		**$3,472,434**
RETURN ON INVESTMENT (TOTAL SAVINGS – TOTAL COSTS)		**$3,392,810**

Forchuk, C., Martin, M-L., Corring, D., Sherman, D., Srivastava, R., Harerimana, B., & Cheng, R. (2019). Cost-effectiveness of the implementation of a transitional discharge model for community integration of psychiatric clients: Practice insights and policy implications. *International Journal of Mental Health*, *48*(3), 236–249. https://doi.org/10.1080/00207411.2019.1649237

From a mental healthcare practice perspective, the present study results support that TDM has the potential for reducing clients' stay in the hospital, and thereby improving healthcare costs. TDM implementation can be most successful when it is leveraged in favour of all parties so that it benefits the clients, hospital staff, and community peer supporters (Forchuk et al., 2013). When these groups work together to successfully implement TDM, both the local hospital and healthcare system as a whole may benefit.

The study results further indicate that TDM provides mental health policy one of the most unique opportunities for effective discharge from hospital to community mental health services. By offering continuous support through bridging staff and community peer supporters, TDM may improve the functional and social well-being of benefitting clients; these are essential factors for an effective discharge from inpatient to community integration (Little et al., 2019).

A systematic review of intervention studies highlighted that the implementation of bridging staff, pre- and post-discharge planning, are effective components for reducing early psychiatric readmissions (Vigod et al., 2013). These TDM-related benefits would be sustained by policy frameworks that support consistency of TDM implementation and its economic and social benefits.

Given the success of TDM in the mental health context, it is worth testing the model with other long-term conditions. Previous research has shown peer support effectiveness in health fields such as cancer care (Legg et al., 2017; Stickel et al., 2015) and people living with long-term illness (Taylor & Bury, 2007). Peer support has consistently been linked with positive results whenever there are chronic and or acute life-altering illnesses (Taylor & Bury, 2007). Peer support also positively impacts on the continuity of care among individuals experiencing psychotic disorders (Belling et al., 2011) and seniors discharged from a hospital emergency department (Eklund et al., 2013).

Limitations

The present study used no control or matched cohort groups that could facilitate objective comparisons of results. Besides, the analyses used only direct costs related to implementation and hospital spending, without accounting for indirect cost (e.g., loss of productivity among participants). Because of these limitations, the study results may be used with caution.

Acknowledgements

The authors would like to express gratitude to all individuals whose contributions have led to the completion of this research project.

Funding

This work was supported by Adopting Research to Improve Care (ARTIC) Project through the Council of Academic Hospitals of Ontario.

15 Supporting Therapeutic Relationships in the Clinical Setting

Mary-Lou Martin

Everyone experiences transition in their lives. Each person's experience is unique and dependent on their capacity for managing transition successfully. Transition, a dynamic and complex process, causes stress and challenges, and sometimes it precipitates vulnerability or a crisis (Martin, 2014).

Discharge from the hospital or a transfer from one program to another are examples of transitions that can be challenging for care recipients. Care providers can support care recipients and plan successful transitions by developing therapeutic relationships and by creating and sustaining specific conditions for success. The transitional discharge model (TDM), developed by Forchuk and colleagues (2005), supports the care recipients' transition from the hospital to the community and involves collaboration, partnerships, and supportive interpersonal relationships (Forchuk, Chan, et al., 1998; Forchuk, Jewell, et al., 1998; Forchuk, Schofield, et al., 1998).

Transitional Discharge Model (TDM)

The TDM incorporates peer and overlapping professional support between hospital and community care providers to create a net of safe and supportive relationships (Forchuk et al., 2005; Forchuk et al., 2013; Forchuk et al., 2020; Forchuk, Jewell, et al., 1998; Forchuk, Martin, Sherman, et al., 2019). This seamless transition of care is an important factor for the care recipient's success. Hospital care providers are involved in the discharge process until the care recipient has established a therapeutic relationship with the community care provider (Forchuk et al., 2007a, 2007b; Forchuk et al., 2013; Forchuk, Chan, et al., 1998; Forchuk, Jewell, et al., 1998; Forchuk, Schofield, et al., 1998).

The TDM has demonstrated positive outcomes for both care recipients with mental health issues and nurses (Coatsworth-Puspoky et al., 2006; Forchuk, Chan, et al., 1998; Forchuk, Jewell, et al., 1998; Forchuk, Martin, Corring, et al., 2019; Forchuk, Schofield, et al., 1998). Care providers have reported perceived value in using the TDM and an increased awareness of community integration strategies (Forchuk et al., 2013; Forchuk, Martin, Sherman, et al., 2019; Forchuk, Schofield, et al., 1998). Care providers and peer support workers want to support care recipients; however, this can only happen if supported by quality work environments and strong leadership.

Work Environment and Leadership

Work environment and leadership are important issues to consider in TDM implementation (Forchuk et al., 2013). To implement the TDM, there must be a culture that can support therapeutic relationships, peer support services, and an overlap between hospital and community care providers. It is important to assess the culture of hospital and community settings for readiness to change.

Leadership plays an important role in ensuring that the TDM is in line with organizational goals and a healthy work environment. Administrators and managers must engage in change management practices and lead policy formulation and implementation. Clinical nurse specialists (CNSs) can provide leadership and assist care providers with implementing the TDM. The availability and stability of on-site care providers (e.g., nurses, social workers) as champions can help sustain the TDM (Forchuk et al., 2007a, 2007b; Forchuk et al., 2013). Champions can support problem-solving and be a resource. Administrators, managers, CNSs, and champions can support others to accept change and demonstrate new behaviours. The work environment and leaders need to support the translation of knowledge and skills into practice and policy.

Practice, Policy, Procedures, and Protocols

Standardized policies facilitate and support effective practice and communication between care providers, care recipients, and peer support workers. The TDM means evolving from traditional policy to evidence-informed policy that reflects transitional care (Martin et al., 2007). It is usual for organizations and care providers to be resistive to change. Therefore, it is important to demonstrate the relevance of the TDM and how it links with practice and positive outcomes. TDM practice, policy, procedures, and protocols must support care transitions, therapeutic relationships, peer support, community integration, and professional development. Policy in hospital and community settings must articulate processes for communicating and protecting privacy and confidentiality.

Health professionals suggest that developing documents to describe the roles of team members and peer support workers are helpful so that roles are co-created and everyone is knowledgeable about expectations (Forchuk, Martin, Sherman, et al., 2019). One role of care providers is to ensure that care recipients are connected in the hospital to peer support workers prior to discharge (Forchuk, Martin, Sherman, et al., 2019). Peer support workers also need policy to address relationships, safety, and supervision (Forchuk et al., 2020).

Staffing and Scheduling

Shift schedules, staffing, and work assignments can be barriers to effective transitional care. The staffing models in hospital settings have not changed much over several decades. Appropriate staffing can be challenged by increased demand for healthcare services and associated healthcare costs. Hospital care providers are assigned shifts for a given planning period; however, depending on the needs of care recipients and care provider resources, the schedule can change shortly before a shift begins. Scheduling and staffing are complex issues that affect care outcomes and satisfaction of care recipients and care providers.

It is important that care providers communicate with care recipients and peer support workers. Care providers working five eight-hour shifts (day, evening, or night shifts) or three 12-hour day and night shifts are more able to develop therapeutic relationships and communicate effectively with care recipients than care providers who work only nights, particularly eight-hour shifts. Staff shortages, part-time care providers, or the wrong type of care provider can also inhibit the development of a therapeutic relationship and be a barrier to the TDM.

Work Assignments and Workload

Continuity in the care provider's assignment should be facilitated. Work assignments must consider the knowledge, skills, competence, and experience of the care provider. Keep in mind that the hospital care provider in the TDM provides care before, during, and after discharge from the hospital.

Care recipients have confirmed the importance of their therapeutic relationships with care providers in the transition from the hospital to the community (Forchuk, Jewell, et al., 1998; Forchuk, Schofield, et al., 1998). Initially, when nurses used the TDM, they identified feeling uncertain when embracing both a hospital and community care role; however, after ten months, they no longer expressed uncertainty (Forchuk, Jewell, et al., 1998; Forchuk, Schofield, et al., 1998). It is important that flexibility be built into patient assignments. The TDM helps support transitional care whereby the nurse and care recipient establish a therapeutic relationship, respect each other, and engage in client-focused care (Forchuk, Jewell, et al., 1998; Forchuk, Schofield, et al., 1998).

Workload issues impact job satisfaction and will be different between settings. Care providers' workload must be reasonable because it can affect quality of care. A barrier to the TDM is care providers who feel burdened and overwhelmed, so it is important to have workload balance (Forchuk et al., 2013). Workload balance must consider transitional care that is happening in the hospital or community, and whether it involves face-to-face contact or contact through technology. Care-provider-to-care-recipient assignments must be planned proactively. For example, the time and distance to meet a care recipient and/or community provider and/ or peer support worker must be measured and recorded to effectively apportion assignments. When hospital or community care providers take vacation, sick time, or a leave of absence, it is important that an alternate care provider who has a relationship with the care recipient step in and provide transitional care.

Communication

Hospital and community care providers, peer support workers, and care recipients must communicate effectively at any time, but particularly during transition. Face-to-face contact with the care recipient is not the only way to do therapeutic work; telephone or video contact can be especially important for routine care or crisis calls. For example, when there is overlap between hospital and community care providers, a care recipient can talk to a familiar care provider from the hospital unit 24/7. The hospital care provider will be able to access documentation and the cost of a phone call will be less than emergency services.

Documentation

Documentation needs to support the TDM to ensure that communication about care recipients, care providers, and peer support workers is recorded (Forchuk et al., 2007b; Forchuk et al., 2013). Many settings implementing the TDM have developed checklists, algorithms, flow sheets, decision sheets, protocols, care pathways, care plans, discharge and transition documents, and forms for transfer, referral, or follow-up. The TDM Toolkit in this book has some examples of these tools.

Documentation needs to reflect the current state and future planning related to the care recipient's situation. For example, care providers are involved in the transfer of information as the care recipient is transitioning to a different setting or level of care. Documentation is ongoing and needs to be available and accessible. It must identify the hospital care provider, community care provider, and peer support worker that is working with the care recipient (Forchuk, Martin, Sherman, et al., 2019).

Electronic health records (EHRs) can be helpful; however, not all institutions have EHRs. These systems provide standardization that can support finding information quickly and facilitate communication between hospital and community services. Each jurisdiction should have legislation that ensures the protection of privacy, confidentiality, and security of information.

Education

Administrative and management support of continuing education and training activities is important to the success of TDM implementation (Forchuk et al., 2007b). Educational strategies for care providers will vary depending on academic preparation and type of provider. Nurses identified that educational support was needed to both attain and support community integration and that experiential learning was the best approach (Forchuk, Schofield, et al., 1998).

The hospital nurses who were transitioning care recipients to the community asked the expert community nurses to accompany them on their community visits and provide feedback (Forchuk, Schofield, et al., 1998). Nurses identified their learning needs as knowledge and skills about their changing roles (Forchuk, Jewell, et al., 1998; Forchuk, Schofield, et al., 1998). Learning needs identified by hospital nurses were focused on community resources, while learning needs identified by public health nurses were focused on clinical management and medications. Both groups of nurses found that when they worked collaboratively, they learned knowledge and skills from each other (Forchuk, Schofield, et al., 1998).

Reynolds et al. (2004) used one training day to teach nurses about the TDM. Training included knowledge about therapeutic relationships, the role of the transitional nurse, and how hospital and community nurses could provide overlapping therapeutic relationships and still work effectively together. They also provided peer support training, which included rules of conduct and relationship boundaries.

Martin and colleagues' (2007) approach to TDM staff education included a learning needs assessment, a literature review, and the expertise of CNSs. TDM implementation was influenced by care providers' abilities to integrate new knowledge from education modules into practice (Martin et al., 2007). Strategies for knowledge integration also included support from the organization and leadership, care providers, care recipients, and peer support workers.

Care providers and peer support workers appreciated having TDM education modules prior to implementation (Forchuk et al., 2013; Holbert et al., 2003). Educational themes included the TDM, best practices, therapeutic relationships, peer support, therapeutic boundaries, discharge planning, telepractice, safety, crisis intervention, and resources (Forchuk et al., 2013). Care providers wanted education offered online and indicated satisfaction with interactive half or full-day workshops and case/person-centered learning (Forchuk et al., 2013). Flexibility is important in teaching approaches, so a variety of learners' needs are met.

Ongoing and updated education about the TDM must be integrated into the orientation and onboarding of care providers. It can also be important to have refreshers. Some units created resource binders with relevant TDM information for care providers.

Posters, postcards, and pamphlets were suggested by care providers as an effective way to share TDM information with care recipients (Forchuk, Martin, Sherman, et al., 2019).

Peer support workers need specialized training in peer support and situation specific training (Forchuk et al., 2020; Forchuk, Martin, Sherman, et al., 2019). The education for peer support workers is described in the Ontario Peer Development Initiative Peer Support Core Essentials Training Program (https://www.opdi.org/news-events/events/traing/opdi-peersupport-core-essentials-training-program).

Technology

Technology can connect people in hospitals, community settings, homes, and workplaces. It has the potential to facilitate communication between the care recipient, peer support worker, and community and hospital care providers. Most healthcare settings have technology; however, many care recipients do not. Therefore, it is important to assess the care recipient's access to and familiarity with technology. What do they currently use and how often? The care recipient may not have a cell phone or a computer or may not be able to afford data on their devices.

Virtual care can complement regular face-to-face visits and enhance transition when people are not able to meet in-person. If the care recipient lives in a rural area, it could mean that travel may be impractical due to distance, time requirements, lack of transportation, and expense. Technology can support education, counselling, and psychotherapy of care recipients, and education, coaching, mentoring, and clinical supervision of care providers and peer support workers.

Conclusion

The TDM is a client-centered, evidence-based practice that involves therapeutic relationships, peer support, and collaborative partnerships in transitional care. This model translates into positive outcomes for care recipients, care providers, peer support workers, costs, and the healthcare system. To implement and sustain the TDM, there must be a foundation of ongoing support that includes a quality work environment and strong leadership in hospital and community clinical settings.

Conclusion

Cheryl Forchuk

The interpersonal therapeutic relationship is foundational to all nursing practice. The Registered Nurses' Association of Ontario (2002/2006) best practice guideline on establishing therapeutic relationships states that in some contexts, like emergency care, the relationship may be in the background to nursing activities, while in other contexts, like mental health or palliative care, it is in the foreground. In mental healthcare, relationships are foundational across all professions.

The early work on therapeutic relationships was pioneered by Dr. Hildegard Peplau who developed a theory that included the client as a partner in care. Peplau's theory highlighted the importance of self-reflection and understanding the relationship as an evolving interpersonal process, the goal of which was to improve the client's health. Dr. Peplau states "…every nurse-patient relationship is an interpersonal situation in which recurring difficulties of everyday living occur," (1952, p. xiii) and later "…every nurse-patient relationship is an opportunity for tackling collaboratively those disagreements in point of view that are inevitable" (1991, p. xi).

Peplau's theory was developed during a very different time. I remember one year we invited Dr. Nora Parker to speak at Hamilton Psychiatric Hospital during nursing week. Dr. Parker was the chair of the graduate department at the Faculty of Nursing at the University of Toronto when I did my master's degree there. She had completed her basic training at (what became) Hamilton Psychiatric Hospital. In her reflections about what psychiatric nursing was like in the few years following World War II, she described a situation where only one physician/psychiatrist was staffed at the hospital and where the director of nursing and the director of the school of nursing served as the only registered nurses, with most programs staffed by nursing students. These were the only staff for about 5,000 patients. She described the period after the war as a time when increasing nursing staff levels was a priority. After graduating from nursing school, Dr. Parker was hired as a head nurse, which she said was not as impressive as it sounded, since she was the only nurse among 100 patients and student nurses. She explained how patient peer support was integral, as people who were healthier helped those in distress. After a couple of years, a second nurse was hired for the ward and she wondered what to do with all the help! So, when Peplau focused only on the nurse–patient relationship, it was for the practical reason that that *was* the staff team.

In the transitional discharge model (TDM), we broaden the emphasis on relationships to include the interprofessional team. Other professions have emerged over the years as healthcare has become more complex and more specialized. It could be argued that all healthcare still depends on relationships. However, in mental healthcare, this argument is quite evident – a client agreeing to take medication has even been found to be dependent on the relationship with the care provider (Kerse et al., 2004).

One of the basic assumptions of both Peplau's work and the TDM is that people heal in relationships. This assumption is not limited to professional relationships, but also includes friends and family. With TDM, we explicitly look at the network of relationships to support a person. This model is consistent with Peplau's theory and brings it forward to current contexts of care.

Although this is the conclusion of the book, there are some important tools in the appendices, including a relationship form that considers both therapeutic and non-therapeutic relationships. With the TDM, hospital staff stay involved until there is a working relationship formed with the community care provider. Therefore, knowing how to recognize a working relationship is important. In some situations, such relationships already exist in the community. Also included are forms that review existing supports prior to discharge.

Appendix
The Transitional Discharge Model Toolkit

This toolkit includes examples of tools developed to assist in implementing the transitional discharge model.

The Relationship Form

The Relationship Form helps assess the current phase of the relationship. This form was originally reported in Forchuk and Brown (1989). At that point, it was used as part of a community mental health program. The Relationship Form at that time reflected the phases of the development of therapeutic relationships as described by Peplau (1952). As we learned in Chapter 6, there are also phases of non-therapeutic relationships. Both therapeutic and non-therapeutic relationships start in the orientation phase (the shaded area on The Relationship Form). Moving left to right from the orientation phase, we see the working phase (subdivided into identification and exploitation) and the resolution phase. If you start in the orientation phase and move to the left, you will see the phases of non-therapeutic relationships. The orientation phase moves to a phase of grappling and struggling and then mutual withdrawal. As well, note that the top part of The Relationship Form reflects client behaviours and the bottom part reflects service provider behaviours.

The phases of the relationship are interlocking and overlapping. Using the check spots in Table A.1, you can tally where the most frequent behaviours occur.

For those wishing to use The Relationship Form as part of research or practice, we would like to hear of this and maintain copyright. Please see the permission form. There is no cost for its use, but we would like to track this.

Table A.1 Phases of the Therapeutic Relationship

Phases of the Therapeutic Relationship

Non-Therapeutic Relationships		←START→		Therapeutic Relationships	
Mutual Withdrawal	Grappling	Orientation	Working Phase		Resolution Phase
			Identification	Exploitation	

Client:

Mutual Withdrawal	Grappling	Orientation	Identification (Working Phase)	Exploitation	Resolution Phase
• forgets appointment/ planned times • cannot recall who nurse/service provider is • unaware if nurse/ service provider is available • content kept superficial • actively avoids nurse/service provider	• frequent changes of topics and approach • increasing frustration • sense of lack of connection • begins to dread meetings	• seeks assistance • conveys educative needs • asks questions • tests parameters • shares preconceptions and expectations due to past experience	• identifies problems • aware of time • responds to help • identifies with service provider • recognizes service provider as a person • explores feelings • fluctuates dependence, independence and interdependence in therapeutic relationship • increases focal attention • changes appearance (for better or worse) • understands purpose of meeting • maintains continuity between sessions (process and content) • testing manoeuvres decrease • increase focal attention	• makes full use of services • identifies new goals • rapid shifts in behaviour; dependent- independent • exploitative behaviour • realistic exploitation • self-directing • develops skills in interpersonal relationships and problem-solving • displays changes in manner of communication (more open, flexible)	• abandons old needs • aspires to new goals • becomes independent of helping person • applies new problem-solving skills • maintains changes in style of communication and interaction • positive changes in view of self • integrates illness • exhibits ability to stand alone

Service Provider:

Mutual Withdrawal	Grappling	Orientation	Identification (Working Phase)	Exploitation	Resolution Phase
• no time for client meetings • client meetings very short if they occur at all • focus on instrumental tasks • decision that client is atypical of usual relationship • avoids client contact	• frequent changes of therapeutic approach • sense of lack of connection • increasing frustration • length of meetings vary • place of meetings vary	• respond to emergency • give parameters of meetings • explain roles • gather data • help client identify problem • help client plan use of community resources and services • reduce anxiety and tension • practice non-directive listening • focus client's energies • clarify preconceptions and expectations	• maintain separate identity • unconditional acceptance • help express needs, feelings • assess and adjust to needs • provide information • provide experiences that diminish feelings of helplessness • do not allow anxiety to overwhelm client • help focus on cues • help client develop responses to cues • use word stimuli	• continue assessment • meet needs as they emerge • understand reason for shifts in behaviour • initiate rehabilitative plans • reduce anxiety • identify positive factors • help plan for total needs • facilitate forward movement of personality • deal with therapeutic impasse	• sustain relationship as long as patient feels necessary • promote family interaction • assist with goal setting • teach preventive measures • utilize community agencies • teach self-care • terminate relationship

Note: Phases Are Overlapping

MW	GR	O	WP	RP

Please mark on the following scale where the check marks are concentrated within the above table. Check lists designed to assist in evaluating phase.

Completed by: _____ **Date:** _____

Peplau, H. E. (1952). *Interpersonal Relations in Nursing.* New York: G.P. Putnam's Sons.
Peplau, H. E. (1973). Audio-tape series. San Antonio, Texas: P.F.S. Productions.
Forchuk, C., & Brown, B. (1989). Establishing A Nurse-Client Relationship. *Journal of Psychosocial Nursing, 27*(2), 30–34.
Forchuk,C., Westwell, J., et al. (2000). The Development Nurse-Client Relationship: Nurses' Perspectives. *Journal of the American Psychiatric Nurses Association, 691,* 3–10.
Copyright revised Cheryl Forchuk 2000.

Staff training

We have found this list of training topics to be helpful for staff. It is helpful for teams to learn the material together and to have peer supporters present. Topics can be covered in a full day retreat or two half-day retreats.

Therapeutic Relationships: From Hospital to Community

Transitional Discharge Model Staff Learning Topics

A learning needs assessment was completed in relation to the multidisciplinary staff's participation in the research project. Training sessions have been developed based on the learning needs identified by multidisciplinary staff.

The training sessions include:

1. INTRODUCTION TO THE *THERAPEUTIC RELATIONSHIPS* TRANSITIONAL DISCHARGE MODEL
2. BEST PRACTICES
3. PEER SUPPORT
4. THERAPEUTIC RELATIONSHIPS: ESTABLISHING, MAINTAINING AND TERMINATING
5. THERAPEUTIC BOUNDARIES
6. TRANSITIONAL PLANNING
7. COMMUNITY PARTNERS AND RESOURCES
8. SAFETY IN THE COMMUNITY
9. CRISIS INTERVENTION
10. TELEPHONE ADVICE

Implementation Tools for Staff

The Transitional Discharge Planning, Step by Step example and Implementing the Transitional Discharge Model of Care: A Staff Checklist (see Figure A.1) were developed during the Council of Academic Hospitals of Ontario study to summarize process.

Transitional Discharge Planning, Step by Step Example

Admission to Hospital

- Client is admitted to hospital.
- Initiate the Transitional Discharge Plan. *The clinical team begins to identify general needs and goals of hospitalization and assess the client's potential "match" with a clinical team member. Ensure a clear and consistent documentation practice is in place, which is accessible to all relevant team members both during and after hospitalization (Refer to the "Transitional Discharge Planning Guide").*
- If a previous therapeutic relationship exists between this client and an inpatient staff, re-establish this relationship. *Remember, the inpatient staff can be from any discipline (e.g., social work, occupational therapy, psychiatry, nursing, spiritual care, recreation, psychology, etc.). Although this is the relationship that will "bridge" the client to the community, each team member will remain a valuable and integral part of the client's inpatient care.*
- As the Bridging Staff, you will begin to establish or re-establish a therapeutic relationship with the client (this may progress quickly or take up to 6-12 months in some cases).

- Evaluate your relationship with the client (Refer to "The Relationship Form"). In addition to your own reflective practice, ask for feedback from team members. Identify and deal with any boundary issues.
- If the relationship is not progressing therapeutically, assess the need for a different Bridging Staff and begin the process of establishing a therapeutic relationship with the client.

During Hospitalization

- Revisit the Transitional Discharge Plan. *Regularly review and update the Transitional Discharge Plan collaboratively with the client to reflect the client's specific needs, goals and strengths. Are goals compatible with personal strengths and resources? Are they realistic and obtainable? Discuss expected time frames and review the Transitional Discharge Plan. Ensure potential community care providers have been identified and discussed. Remember that transitional discharge planning involves family members and other non-clinical supports that are important to the client's recovery and well-being.*
- Continue the "working phase" of your relationship and explore the needs, goals and values of the client and their identified/perceived supports (e.g. family, friends, cultural or spiritual community, etc.). *Reflect on what behaviours demonstrate the working phase of your relationship. Identify and work through any boundary issues.*
- Remind the client that you will continue to work with them until they feel comfortable with the community care provider and are ready to terminate the relationship with you. *Ensure your manager/supervisor/clinical team supports your flexible role with the client post-hospitalization. Remember that clients may be unfamiliar with ongoing post-hospital support from inpatient staff and may require frequent reminders of your availability and frequent checks on potential boundary issues.*
- Evaluate your relationship with the client (refer to The Relationship Form). *Is your relationship progressing? What is facilitating or hindering the progress of your relationship? What behaviours indicate this? Check for boundary issues and get feedback from trusted team members.*
- Assess whether the client perceives themself as "lonely". *Remember that the transitional discharge model is most effective with those who identify themselves as lonely.*
- Introduce the idea of peer support to the client as soon as possible or appropriate. Discuss the role and benefits of a peer supporter. If the client is willing, contact the peer support coordinator of your local consumer group and facilitate introductions between the peer volunteer and the client, or the client may wish to contact the consumer group themself. *Remember that the consumer group needs time to find a suitable trained peer volunteer, so start this process well before the anticipated time that the client will leave hospital.*
- Based on the client's perceived needs and goals and preferences, establish who the community care provider (CCP) will be in the client's community. *Remember, the CCP could be a family physician, nurse practitioner, psychologist, psychiatrist, community case manager, ACT member, social worker, therapist, etc. The CCP could be someone who has a well-established therapeutic relationship with the client or could be someone new. Also remember, the client's "community" is not simply a geographic location, but a supportive environment where the client has access to the supports and resources that are identified as meaningful and important to that client's recovery after hospitalization.*
- Facilitate an introductory meeting where you, the CCP, and the client discuss expectations, roles, and transitional planning. *It is vital to be clear with the CCP about your ongoing involvement after the client leaves hospital and that the client will decide when they have developed a therapeutic relationship with the CCP and no longer need your bridging services. It is also important to discuss with the CCP the role of peer support during transition. Remember that this meeting could be held in hospital but may be more effective or appropriate in the client's*

community. Since the CCP may not be familiar with the transitional discharge model, it may be helpful to leave a brief summary of the transitional discharge model with the CCP (Refer to Summary). Invite the CCP to participate in transitional planning meetings.

- Evaluate your relationship with the client (refer to The Relationship Form). *How is the relationship progressing? How is the transitional discharge planning process affecting this relationship? What have you observed about the beginning relationship between the client and the CCP?*
- Evaluate the Transitional Discharge Plan with the inpatient team, client, and CCP. *Ensure the Transitional Discharge Plan addresses all aspects of a supportive post-hospital environment (refer to The Transitional Discharge Planning Guide), and ensure the Bridger, CCP, and client are clear about their roles and responsibilities. Remember, with the client's consent, the peer support worker can be involved in transitional discharge planning.*

After the Client Leaves Hospital

- When the client leaves the hospital, ensure that they are aware of the parameters around your continued contact. *Will you be available to visit/call the hospital or the client's home? When is your first contact? Is there an alternate bridging staff who can respond to the client if needed?*
- Communicate your continued contact clearly! *Ensure you document every contact in a chart or form that is readily accessible. You may need to make arrangements to keep the inpatient chart or a similar record on the ward until bridging is complete. Remember, many clinicians fail to document those information-seeking phone calls, or short, reassuring contacts that make a big difference to clients. Ensure your time and expertise are given proper credit and remember that post-hospitalization contacts are an extension of your continued therapeutic relationship, and therefore* require *proper documentation. Document the nature and frequency of your contacts as well as any advice given. Also, update the CCP regularly regarding your continued contact – the CCP should know how to reach you and reciprocate and inform you of their client contacts.*
- Regularly assess your therapeutic relationship (refer to The Relationship Form). *Reflect on the behaviours you and the client are displaying and note whether you are still in the working phase or whether you are moving toward (or in) the termination phase. Ask the client how they perceive their relationship with the CCP. Ensure that along with exchanging information with the CCP, you and the CCP discuss how your respective relationships with the client are progressing.*
- According to the Transitional Discharge Plan, assess whether goals are being met, and how the client is progressing toward these goals. *Is the client becoming more independent? Seeking out different resources? Relying less on you for support and more on the CCP? Making social connections (perhaps through the peer supporter) and using community resources? Calling or contacting you infrequently?*
- Ask the client whether they feel your bridging relationship is still meeting identified needs. If so, sustain the relationship for as long as the client feels necessary. If not, begin terminating your relationship (refer to Establishing, Maintaining and Terminating the Therapeutic Relationship). *Remember, any changes in follow-up (i.e., new CCP) during this time would require the Bridger to continue working with the client until a therapeutic working relationship has been established with the new CCP.*
- Document the completion of the Transitional Discharge Plan and the termination of your involvement. *Ensure the CCP, inpatient team, your supervisor, and any other relevant people are fully aware of the termination of your bridging service.*

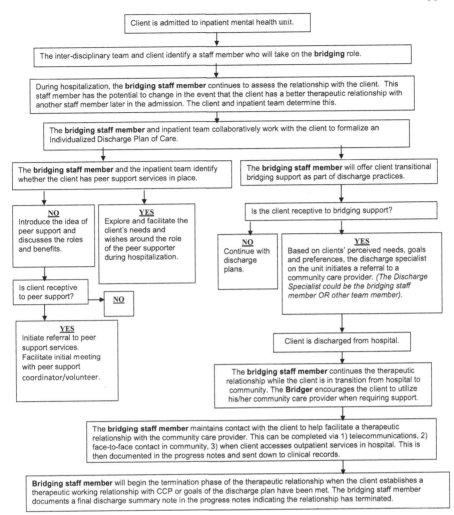

Figure A.1 Implementing the Transitional Discharge Model of Care: A Staff Checklist.

- Reflect on your bridging experience. *Review the challenges and successes of your role, your new learning, and seek feedback from team members/supervisors. Act as a resource for new Bridging Staff and ensure your new skills and work effort are given credit in your performance appraisal, continuing education requirements, and work measurement.*

Client Information

The brochure entitled "Program Information: Transitional Discharge Model" (see Figure A.2) is an example developed at the Hôpital Montfort and Psychiatric Survivors of Ottawa that can be given upon admission to introduce people to the concept of peer support. The hospital is French but also had this English version. Also included is an example of information given at one of the sites to clients at discharge.

How the Program works

The Transitional Discharge Model
(TDM); Project components:

1. **Peer Support (PSO):** Support from
   a person/Peer Supporter who has
   experienced a mental illness, is
   living successfully in the community,
   and has completed a peer training
   program. The support includes
   regular contact on a schedule that
   suits both parties, for the purpose of
   providing social support and shared
   learning from the experience of
   someone who has lived through a
   similar transition.

2. **Hospital Staff Support:** Continued
   support from a staff person from the
   hospital program, or a community
   program until a therapeutic
   relationship has been established or
   re-established with a community
   mental health care provider.

 Psychiatric
Survivors
of Ottawa

 Hôpital
Montfort

A partnership between Psychiatric Survivors
of Ottawa and Montfort Hospital

Program Information

Transitional
Discharge Model

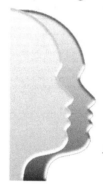

*"Peer Support has a healing
power that can lift, guide and
root people who have mental*

Progress Report to the Change Foundation.
www.psychiatricsurvivors.org/Final_Report.pdf

CAHO
Council of Academic Hospitals of Ontario

*Sharing
the
Recovery
journey*

What are the benefits of the Transitional Discharge Model?

- Supports the successful
  transition from hospital to
  the community for people
  diagnosed with a mental
  illness.

- Promotes a reduction in
  the length of stay and
  readmission rates for
  people being discharged
  from psychiatric beds.

- The model is based on
  therapeutic relationships
  and supports the
  successful community
  integration of people with
  mental health challenges.

*A treatment plan based on hope
is essential. People cannot
recover without hope."*
--Progress Report to the Change Foundation
www.psychiatricsurvivors.org/Final_Report.
pdf

Other Benefits

By connecting to a peer supporter,
you will experience a respectful,
trusting, non-judgmental
relationship with someone who
understands the recovery journey.

You will have the chance to take
part in activities that you enjoy with
the peer supporter. You may feel
more hopeful when you hear about
how the peer supporter has
experienced recovery.

By participating in this project, you
will help Psychiatric Survivors of
Ottawa and the Montfort Hospital
continue to help promote mental
health recovery. Your participation
will not only benefit you but may
inspire others to access the
Transitional Discharge Model.

Have you faced challenges to your mental health?

Imagine what it would have been
like if you'd had a peer supporter
to call on, someone who had
gone through the mental health
system and was willing to listen
to your story; a confidant who
could offer encouragement as
you slowly stepped back into
society; someone to reassure
you that you're not alone.
Hospital staff will assist you in
accessing the Transitional
Discharge Model.
Once you've joined the program,
PSO will match you with a peer
supporter.

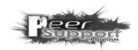

Figure A.2 How the Program works.

Transitional Discharge Planning – Information for Clients

BRIDGING STAFF

Name of Bridging Staff_____

Phone Number_____

Alternate Bridging Staff_____

Phone Number_____

Other Information:

COMMUNITY CARE PROVIDER

Name of Community Care Provider_____

Agency_____

Location_____

Phone Number_____

Other Information:

PEER SUPPORT WORKER

Name of Peer Support Worker_____

Agency_____

Phone Number/Contact Information_____

Other Information:

HOUSING

Address_____

Phone Number_____

Landlord or Contact Person at Residence_____

Directions or Bus Route_____

Other Information:

SOCIAL/RECREATIONAL

Regular Social Activities:

(Date, Time, Activity, Special Instructions, etc.)

MON	TUES	WED	THURS	FRI	SAT	SUN

OTHER ACTIVITIES_____

FAMILY

Name and Relationship_____

Home Phone Number_____

Work Phone Number_____

Other Information:

WORK/SCHOOL/VOLUNTEER ACTIVITIES

Agency_____

Phone Number_____

Contact Person_____

What to Do If I Can't Attend: _____

Other Information:

REGULAR WORK ACTIVITIES:

(Date, Time, Activity, Special Instructions, etc.)

MON	TUES	WED	THURS	FRI	SAT	SUN

OTHER_____

FINANCES
Budget Information (e.g., Weekly Budget, Regular Bills or Expenses):

Name and Location of Bank_____

Name and Phone Number of Bank Representative_____

Public Trustee (IF APPLICABLE) Name_____

Public Trustee Phone Number_____

What to do if I don't have enough money:

Food Bank (Location)_____

Amity/Goodwill Clothing Shop_____

MEDICAL CARE

Name of Family Doctor/Nurse Practitioner/

Medical Clinic_____

Phone Number_____

Location_____

Hours of Service_____

WHAT TO DO IF I HAVE A MEDICAL CONCERN AFTER HOURS:

Location of Nearest Walk-In Medical Clinic_____

Location of Nearest Hospital Emergency Department_____

Additional Phone Numbers (e.g. TeleHealth)_____

Dentist Name and Phone Number_____

Current Medications:

Name & Location of Pharmacy_____

Phone Number of Pharmacy_____

PSYCHIATRIC CARE

Name of Psychiatrist_____

Phone Number and Location_____

WHAT TO DO IF I HAVE URGENT CONCERNS ABOUT MY MENTAL HEALTH OR
SAFETY:

OTHER SUPPORTS

Spiritual Advisor_____

OTHERS (e.g., Art Group, Schizophrenia Society, Irish-Canadians Social Club, Probation
Officer, Alcoholics Anonymous)

_____

OTHER IMPORTANT INFORMATION

e.g., Community College Continuing Education Department, Volunteer Organizations, Animal Shelter, Neighbour(s), Red Cross Volunteer Drivers

_____

_____

_____

_____

_____

_____

MY GOALS

(Also refer to copy of the Transitional Discharge Plan, if available)

PLANNED MEETINGS/APPOINTMENTS
OR TELEPHONE CONTACTS

DATE	TIME	PERSON(S)	LOCATION	GOALS

Copyright Acknowledgements

Cover Art: Written permission to use cover art, *The Bridge*, obtained from creator Norma Jean Kelly.

Chapter 1: Some materials reprinted from Forchuk, C. (1993). *Hildegard E. Peplau: Interpersonal nursing theory*. SAGE Publications, Inc. Rights reverted from SAGE Publications, Inc. back to Cheryl Forchuk in January 2004.

Reprinted with permission from original author Cheryl Forchuk.

The Relationship Form: Forchuk, C., & Brown, B. E. (1989). Establishing a nurse-client relationship. *Journal of Psychosocial Nursing*, *27*(2), 30–34. https://doi.org/10.3928/0279-3695-19890201-10

Reprinted with permission from publisher SLACK, Inc.

Chapter 2: Forchuk, C. (1994). The orientation phase of the nurse-client relationship: Testing Peplau's theory. *Journal of Advanced Nursing*, *20*(3), 532–537. https://doi.org/10.1111/j.1365-2648.1994.tb02392.x

Reprinted with permission from publisher John Wiley and Sons.

Chapter 4: Forchuk, C., Westwell, J., Martin, M.-L., Bamber-Azzapardi, W., Kosterewa-Tolman, D., & Hux, M. (1998). Factors influencing movement of chronic psychiatric patients from the orientation to the working phase of the nurse-client relationship on an inpatient unit. *Perspectives in Psychiatric Care*, *34*(1), 36–44. https://doi.org/10.1111/j.1744-6163.1998.tb00998.x

Reprinted with permission from publisher John Wiley and Sons.

Chapter 6: Forchuk, C., Westwell, J., Martin, M.-L., Bamber-Azzapardi, W., Kosterewa-Tolman, D., & Hux, M. (2000). The developing nurse-client relationship: Nurses' perspectives. *Journal of the American Psychiatric Nurses Association*, *6*(1), 3–10. https://doi.org/10.1177%2F107839030000600102

Reprinted with permission from publisher SAGE Publishing, Inc.

Chapter 11: Forchuk, C., Martin, M.-L., Chan, L., & Jensen, E. (2005). Therapeutic relationships: From psychiatric hospital to community. *Journal of Psychiatric and Mental Health Nursing*, *12*(5), 556–564. https://doi.org/10.1111/j.1365-2850.2005.00873.x

Reprinted with permission from publisher John Wiley and Sons.

Chapter 12: Forchuk, C., Solomon, M., & Virani, T. (2016). Peer support: An important part of transitional discharge. *Healthcare Quarterly*, *18*(special issue), 32–36. https://doi.org/10.12927/hcq.2016.24480

Reprinted with permission from publisher Longwoods Publishing.

References

Adair, C., McDougall, M., Beckie, A., Joyce, A., Mitton, C., Wild, C., Gordon, A., & Costigan, N. (2003). History and measurement of continuity of care in mental health services and evidence of its role in outcomes. *Psychiatric Services*, *54*(10), 1351–1356. https://doi.org/10.1176/appi.ps.54. 10.1351

Alberta Health Services. (n.d.). *Attitudes and assumptions.* https://www.albertahealthservices.ca/web apps/elearning/TIC/Mod01/story_content/external_files/AttitudesAssumptions.pdf

Altman, H. (1983). Effects of empathy, warmth and genuineness in the initial counselling interview. *Counsellor Education and Supervision*, *2*, 225–228. https://doi.org/10.1002/j.1556-6978.1973.tb01 555.x

Altwalbeh, D., Mousa Khamaiseh, A., & Algaralleh, A. (2018). Self-reported empathy among nursing students at a university in Jordan. *The Open Nursing Journal*, *12*, 255–263. http://dx.doi.org/10.2174 /1874434601812010255

AMA Principles of Medical Ethics. (2019). *Principles of medical ethics.* https://www.ama-assn.org/deliv ering-care/ethics/code-medical-ethics-overview

Anderson, K., & Handelsman, M. (2010). *Ethics for psychotherapists and counselors: A proactive approach.* Wiley-Blackwell.

Anderson, M., & Perrin, A. (2017). *Tech adoption climbs among older adults.* https://www.pewresearch .org/internet/2017/05/17/tech-adoption-climbs-among-older-adults/

Ardito, R. B., & Rabellino, D. (2011). Therapeutic alliance and outcome of psychotherapy: Historical excursus, measurements, and prospects for research. *Frontiers in Psychology*, *2*(270). https://doi.org /10.3389/fpsyg.2011.00270

Austin, W., Bergum, V., Nuttgens, S., & Peternelj-Taylor, C. (2006). A re-visioning of boundaries in professional helping relationships: Exploring other metaphors. *Ethics & Behavior*, *16*(2), 77–94. https ://doi.org/10.1207/s15327019eb1602_1

Austin, W., Peternelj-Taylor, C. A., Kunyk, D., & Boyd, M. A. (Eds.). (2013). *Psychiatric & mental health nursing for Canadian practice* (4th ed.). Lippincott Williams & Wilkins.

Australian Government Department of Health. (2010). *Principles of recovery oriented mental health practice.* https://www1.health.gov.au/internet/publications/publishing.nsf/Content/mental-pubs-i -nongov-toc~mental-pubs-i-nongov-pri

Baca, M. (2009). Sexual boundaries: Are they common sense? *Journal for Nurse Practitioners*, *5*(7), 500–505. https://doi.org/10.1016/j.nurpra.2009.04.016

Ballatt, J., & Campling, P. (2011). *Intelligent kindness: Reforming the culture of healthcare.* Royal College of Psychiatrists.

Barnett, J. E. (2014). Sexual feelings and behaviors in the psychotherapy relationship: An ethic perspective. *Journal of Clinical Psychology*, *70*(2), 170–181. https://doi.org/10.1002/jclp.22068

Barrett, M. S., & Gershkovich, M. (2014). Computers and psychotherapy: Are we out of a job? *Psychotherapy*, *51*(2), 220–223. https://psycnet.apa.org/doi/10.1037/a0032408

Baum, F. (2007). Therapists' responses to treatment termination: An inquiry into the variables that contribute to therapists' experiences. *Clinical Social Work Journal*, *35*(2), 97–106. https://doi.org/10 .1007/s10615-006-0066-0

Baum, F., MacDougall, C., & Smith, D. (2006). Participatory action research. *Journal of Epidemiology & Community Health, 60*(10), 854–857. http://dx.doi.org/10.1136/jech.2004.028662

Beauchamp, T. L., & Childress, J. F. (2012). *Principles of medical ethics* (7th ed.). Oxford University Press.

Beck, A. (1976). *Cognitive therapy and emotional disorders.* International Universities Press Inc.

Beck, A., Epstein, N., Brown, G., & Steer, R. (1988). An inventory for measuring clinical anxiety: Psychometric properties. *Journal of Clinical and Consulting Psychology, 56*, 893–897. https://doi.org /10.1037//0022-006x.56.6.893

Belling, R., Whittock, M., McLaren, S., Burns, T., Catty, J., Jones, I. R., Rose, D., Wykes, T., & ECHO Group. (2011). Achieving continuity of care: Facilitators and barriers in community mental health teams. *Implementation Science, 6*(1), 23. https://doi.org/10.1186/1748-5908-6-23

Berkman, C. S., Turner, S. G., Cooper, M., Polnerow, D., & Swartz, M. (2000). Sexual contact with clients: Assessment of social workers' attitudes and educational preparation. *Social Work, 45*(3), 223–235. https://doi.org/10.1093/sw/45.3.223

Black, S. C. (2017). To cross or not to cross: Boundaries in psychological practice. *Journal of the Australian & New Zealand Student Services Association, 25*(1), 62–71. https://janzssa.scholasticahq. com/article/1339-to-cross-or-not-to-cross-ethical-boundaries-in-psychological-practice

Bolsinger, J., Jaeger, M., Hoff, P., & Theodoridou, A. (2020). Challenges and opportunities in building and maintaining a good therapeutic relationship in acute psychiatric settings: A narrative review. *Frontiers of Psychiatry, 10*(965). https://dx.doi.org/10.3389%2Ffpsyt.2019.00965

Borys, D., & Pope, K. S. (1989). Dual relationships between therapist and client: A national study of psychologists, psychiatrists, and social workers. *Professional Psychology: Research & Practice, 20*(5), 283–293. https://psycnet.apa.org/doi/10.1037/0735-7028.20.5.283

Bove, L. (2019). Empathy for service: Benefits, unintended consequences and future research agendas. *Journal of Services Marketing, 33*(1), 31–43, https://doi.org/10.1108/JSM-10-2018-0289

Brandt, P. A., & Weinert, C. (1981). The PRQ - A social support measure. *Nursing Research, 30*(5), 271–280. https://doi.org/10.1097/00006199-198109000-00007

Brito-Pons, G., Campos, D., & Cebolla, A. (2018). Implicit or explicit compassion? Effects of compassion cultivation training and comparison with mindfulness-based stress reduction. *Mindfulness, 9*(5), 1494–1508. https://psycnet.apa.org/doi/10.1007/s12671-018-0898-z

Brooten, D., Brown, L. P., Munro, B. H., York, R., Cohen, S. M., Roncoli, M., & Hollingsworth, A. (1988). Early discharge and specialist transitional care. *Journal of Nursing Scholarship, 20*(2), 64–68. https://doi.org/10.1111/j.1547-5069.1988.tb00032.x

Brooten, D., & Duffin, N. M. (1999). Transitional environments. In A. S. Hinshaw, S. L. Feetham, & J. L. F. Shaver (Eds.), *Handbook of clinical nursing research* (pp. 641–653). SAGE Publications Ltd.

Brown, B., Crawford, P., Gilbert, P., Gilbert, J., & Gale, C. (2014). Practical compassions: Repertoires of practice and compassion talk in acute mental healthcare. *Sociology of Health & Illness, 36*(3), 383–399. https://doi.org/10.1111/1467-9566.12065

Browne, G., Arpin, K., Corey, P., Fitch, M., & Gafni, A. (1990). Individual correlates of health services utilization and the cost of poor adjustment to chronic illness. *Medical Care, 28*(1), 43–58. https://doi .org/10.1097/00005650-199001000-00006

Buckman, R. (2010). *Practical plans for difficult conversations in medicine: Strategies that work in breaking bad news.* Johns Hopkins University Press.

Cameron, S. K., Rodgers, J., & Dagnan, D. (2018). The relationship between the therapeutic alliance and clinical outcomes in cognitive behaviour therapy for adults with depression: A meta-analytic review. *Clinical Psychology & Psychotherapy, 25*(3), 446–456. https://doi.org/10.1002/cpp.2180

Canadian Institute for Health Information. (2015). *Canadian institute for health information annual report 2012–2013.* https://secure.cihi.ca/estore/productSeries.htm?pc=PCC241

Canadian Internet Registration Authority. (2018). *The gap between us: Perspectives on building a better online Canada.* https://www.cira.ca/resources/state-internet/report/gap-between-us-perspectives-build ing-a-better-online-canada

Carter, C. S., Bartal, I. B. A., & Porges, E. C. (2017). The roots of compassion: An evolutionary and neurobiological perspective. In E. M. Seppala, E. S. Thomas, S. L. Brown, M. C. Worline, C. D.

Cameron, & J. R. Doty (Eds.), *The Oxford handbook of compassionate science* (pp. 173–208). Oxford University Press.

Carver, E., & Hughes, J. (1990). The significance of empathy. In R. C. MacKay, J. R. Hughes, & E. J. Carver (Eds.), *Empathy in the helping relationship* (pp. 13–27). Springer.

Cassell, J. W. (2002). Compassion. In C. R. Snyder & S. J. Lopez (Eds.), *Handbook of positive psychology* (pp. 433–445). Oxford University Press.

Centre for Addiction and Mental Health. (n.d.). *Stigma*. https://www.camh.ca/en/health-info/guides-and -publications/stigma

Cheng, T. C., Lo, C. C., & Womack, B. G. (2019). Working alliances promote desirable outcomes: A study of case management in the state of Alabama in the USA. *British Journal of Social Work, 1*(1), 147–162. https://doi.org/10.1093/bjsw/bcy030

Chichirez, C. M., & Purcărea, V. L. (2018). Interpersonal communication in healthcare. *Journal of Medicine and Life, 11*(2), 119–122.

Chierchia, G., & Singer, T. (2017). The neuroscience of compassion and empathy and their link to prosocial motivation and behavior. In J.-C. Dreher & L. Tremblay (Eds.), *Decision neuroscience – An integrative perspective* (pp. 247–257). Elsevier. http://hdl.handle.net/11858/00-001M-0000-002B-2454-0

Chilale, H. K., Silungwe, N. D., Gondwe, S., & Masulani-Mwale, C. (2017). Clients and carers perception of mental illness and factors that influence help-seeking: Where they go first and why. *International Journal of Social Psychiatry, 63*(5), 418–425. https://doi.org/10.1177/0020764017709848

Chow, S. L. (1996). *Statistical significance*. SAGE Publications Ltd.

Coatsworth-Puspoky, R., Forchuk, C., & Ward-Griffin, C. (2006). Peer support relationships: An unexplored interpersonal process in mental health. *Journal of Psychiatric and Mental Health Nursing, 13*(5), 490–497. https://doi.org/10.1111/j.1365-2850.2006.00970.x

Cohen, J. (1988). *Statistical power analysis for the behavioral sciences* (2nd ed.). Lawrence Erlbaum Associates, Publishers.

Coleman, E. A., & Berenson, R. A. (2004). Lost in transition: Challenges and opportunities for improving the quality of transitional care. *Annals of Internal Medicine*, 141(7), 533–536. https://doi.org/10.7326 /0003-4819-141-7-200410050-00009

College of Nurses of Ontario. (2006). *Therapeutic nurse-client relationship*. Author. https://www.cno .org/globalassets/docs/prac/41033_therapeutic.pdf

Cooper, A., & Inglehearn, A. (2015). Perspectives: Managing professional boundaries and staying safe in digital spaces. *Journal of Nursing Research, 20*(7), 625–633. https://doi.org/10.1177%2F174498711 5604066

Council of Academic Hospitals of Ontario (CAHO). (n.d.). *The transitional discharge model: People-centred, peer-supported project impactful for both system and clients.* http://caho-hospitals.com/the-transitional-discharge-model-people-centred-peer-supported-project-impactful-for-both-system-an d-clients/#:~:text=System%20and%20Clients-,The%20Transitional%20Discharge%20Model%3A %20People%2DCentred%2C%20Peer%2DSupported,for%20Both%20System%20and%20Clients &text=It%20seeks%20to%20enhance%20the,people%20with%20a%20mental%20illness

Curtis, L. C., & Hodge, M. (1994). Old standards, new dilemmas: Ethics and boundaries in community support services. *Psychosocial Rehabilitation Journal, 18*(2), 13–33. https://psycnet.apa.org/doi/10 .1037/h0095519

Dalgin, R. S., Dalgin, M. H., & Metzger, S. J. (2018). A longitudinal analysis of the influence of a peer run warm line phone service on psychiatric recovery. *Community Mental Health Journal, 54*(4), 376–382. https://doi.org/10.1007/s10597-017-0161-4

Davidson, L., Chinman, M., Kloos, B., Weingarten, R., Stayner, D., & Tebes, J. K. (1999). Peer support among individuals with severe mental illness: A review of the evidence. *Clinical Psychology: Science and Practice, 6*(2), 165–187. https://doi.org/10.1093/clipsy.6.2.165

Davidson, L., Shahar, G., Strayner, D. A., Chinman, M., Rakfeldt, J., & Tebes, J. K. (2004). Supported socialization for people with psychiatric disabilities: Lessons from a randomized controlled trial. *Journal of Community Psychology, 32*(4), 453–477. https://doi.org/10.1002/jcop.20013

Dekker, J., Theunissen, J., Van, R., Kikkert, M., van der Post, L., Zoeteman, J., & Peen, J. (2013). Are long-term psychiatric patients causing more crisis consultations outside office hours in mental health care? *International Journal of Social Psychiatry*, *59*(6), 555–560. https://doi.org/10.1177 /0020764012445259

DeLucia, P. R., Harold, S. A., & Tang, Y. (2013). Innovation in technology-aided psychotherapy through human factors/ergonomics: Toward a collaborative approach. *Journal of Contemporary Psychotherapy*, *43*(4), 253–260. https://doi.org/10.1007/s10879-013-9238-8

Desai, M., & Rosenheck, R. (2003). Trend in discharge disposition, mortality and service use among long-stay psychiatric patients in the 1990s. *Psychiatric Services*, *54*(4), 542–548. https://doi.org/10 .1176/appi.ps.54.4.542

Diehr, P., Martin, D. C., Koepell, T., & Cheadle, A. (1995). Breaking the matches in a paired t-test for community interventions when the number of pairs is small. *Statistics in Medicine*, *14*(13), 1491– 1504. https://doi.org/10.1002/sim.4780141309

Dinc, L., & Gastmans, C. (2012). Trust and trustworthiness in nursing: An argument-based literature review. *Nursing Inquiry*, *19*(3), 223–237. https://doi.org/10.1111/j.1440-1800.2011.00582.x

Dinc, L., & Gastmans, C. (2013). Trust in nurse-patient relationships: A literature review. *Nursing Ethics*, *20*(5), 501–516. https://doi.org/10.1177/0969733012468463

Donner, A., Birkett, N., & Buck, C. (1981). Randomization by cluster: Sample size requirements and analysis. *American Journal of Epidemiology*, *114*(6), 906–914. https://doi.org/10.1093/oxfordjourn als.aje.a113261

Donner, A., & Klar, N. (1994). Cluster randomization trials in epidemiology: Theory and application. *Journal of Statistical Planning and Inference*, *42*(1–2), 37–56. https://doi.org/10.1016/0378-3758(9 4)90188-0

Doser, K., & Norup, A. (2016). Caregiver burden in Danish family members of patients with severe brain injury: The chronic phase. *Brain Injury*, *30*(3), 334–342. https://doi.org/10.3109/02699052.2015.11 14143

Drake, R. E., Goldman, H. H., Leff, H. S., Lehman, A. F., Dixon, L., Mueser, K. T., Torrey, W. C. (2001). Implementing evidence-based practices in routing mental health service settings. *Psychiatric Services*, *52*(2), 79–182. https://doi.org/10.1176/appi.ps.52.2.179

Drebing, C. E., Reilly, E., Henze, K. T., Kelly, M., Russo, A., Smolinsky, J., Gorman, J., & Penk, W. E. (2018). Using peer support groups to enhance community integration of veterans in transition. *Psychological Services*, *15*(2), 135–145. https://doi.org/10.1037/ser0000178

Drury, L. (2008). From homeless to housed: Caring for people in transition. *Journal of Community Health Nursing*, *25*(2), 91–105. https://doi.org/10.1080/07370010802017109

Dziopa, F., & Ahern, K. (2009). Three different ways mental health nurses develop quality therapeutic relationships. *Issues in Mental Health Nursing*, *30*(1), 14–22. https://doi.org/10.1080/01612840802 500691

Easter, A., Pollock, M., Pope, L. G., Wisdom, J. P., & Smith, T. E. (2016). Perspectives of treatment providers and clients with serious mental illness regarding effective therapeutic relationships. *Journal of Behavioral Health Services & Research*, *43*(3), 341–353. https://doi.org/10.1007/s11414-01 5-9492-5

Easterbrook, C. J., & Meehan, T. (2017). The therapeutic relationship and cognitive behavioural therapy: A case study of an adolescent girl with depression. *The European Journal of Counselling Psychology*, *6*(1), 1–24. https://doi.org/10.5964/ejcop.v6i1.85

Eklund, K., Wilhelmson, K., Gustafsson, H., Landahl, S., & Dahlin-Ivanoff, S. (2013). One-year outcome of frailty indicators and activities of daily living following the randomised controlled trial; "Continuum of care for frail older people". *BMC Geriatrics*, *13*(76). https://doi.org/10.1186/1471-2318-13-76

Elliott, R., Bohart, A. C., Watson, J. C., & Murphy, D. (2018). Therapist empathy and client outcome: An updated meta-analysis. *Psychotherapy*, *55*(4), 399–410. https://doi.org/10.1037/pst0000175

Ellis, A. (1962). *Reason and emotion in psychotherapy*. Citadel Press.

Epstein, R. S. (1994). *Keeping boundaries: Maintaining safety and integrity in the psychotherapeutic process*. American Psychiatric Pub.

Eriksson, I., & Nilsson, K. (2008). Preconditions needed for establishing a trusting relationship during health counselling - An interview study. *Journal of Clinical Nursing*, *17*(17), 2352–2359. https://doi .org/10.1111/j.1365-2702.2007.02265.x

Farhall, J., Trauer, T., Newton, R., & Cheung, P. (2003). Minimizing adverse effects on patients of involuntary relation from long-stay wards to community residences. *Psychiatric Services, 54*(7), 1022–1027. https://doi.org/10.1176/appi.ps.54.7.1022

Fazio, R. H. (1986). How do attitudes guide behavior? In R. M. Sorrentino & E. T. Higgins (Eds.), *Handbook of motivation and cognition: Foundations of social behavior* (pp. 204–243). Guilford Press.

Felton, C. J., Stastny, P., Shern, D. L., Blanch, A., Donahue, S. A., Knight, E., & Brown, C. (1995). Consumers as peer specialists on intensive case management teams: Impact on client outcomes. *Psychiatric Services, 46*(10), 1037–1040. https://doi.org/10.1176/ps.46.10.1037

Feo, R., Rasmussen, P., Wiechula, R., Conroy, T., & Kitson, A. (2017). Developing effective and caring nurse-patient relationships. *Nursing Standard, 31*(28), 54–63. https://doi.org/10.7748/ns.2017.e10735

Forchuk, C. (1991). Reconceptualizing the environment of the individual with a chronic mental illness. *Issues in Mental Health Nursing, 12*(2), 159–170. https://doi.org/10.3109/01612849109040511

Forchuk, C. (1992a). The orientation phase of the nurse-client relationship: How long does it take? *Perspectives in Psychiatric Care, 28*(4), 7–10. https://doi.org/10.1111/j.1744-6163.1992.tb00384.x

Forchuk, C. (1992b). *The orientation phase of the nurse-client relationship: Testing Peplau's theory.* Unpublished doctoral dissertation, Wayne State University.

Forchuk, C. (1993). *Hildegard E. Peplau: Interpersonal nursing theory.* SAGE Publications Ltd.

Forchuk, C. (1994). The orientation phase of the nurse-client relationship: Testing Peplau's theory. *Journal of Advanced Nursing, 20*(3), 532–537. https://doi.org/10.1111/j.1365-2648.1994.tb02392.x

Forchuk, C. (1995). Uniqueness in the nurse-client relationship. *Archives of Psychiatric Nursing, 9*, 34–39. https://doi.org/10.1016/S0883-9417(95)80015-8

Forchuk, C., Beaton, S., Crawford, L., Ide, L., Voorberg, N., & Bethune, J. (1986). *A marriage between Peplau's theory and case management instrument development.* [Oral Paper]. Nursing Theories Congress, Ryerson College, Toronto, ON.

Forchuk, C., Beaton, S., Crawford, L., Ide, L.,Voorberg, N., & Bethune, J. (1989). Incorporating Peplau's theory and case management. *Journal of Psychosocial Nursing, 27*(2), 35–38.

Forchuk, C., & Brown, B. E. (1989). Establishing a nurse-client relationship. *Journal of Psychosocial Nursing, 27*(2), 30–34. https://doi.org/10.3928/0279-3695-19890201-10

Forchuk, C., Chan, L., Schofield, R., Martin, M. L., Sircelj, M., Woodcox, V., Valledor, T., Jewell, J., & Overby, B. (1998). Bridging the discharge process. *Canadian Nurse, 94*(3), 22–26.

Forchuk, C., Jewell, J., Schofield, R., Sircelj, M., & Valledor, T. (1998). From hospital to community: Bridging therapeutic relationships. *Journal of Psychiatric and Mental Health Nursing, 5*(3), 197–202. https://doi.org/10.1046/j.1365-2850.1998.00125.x

Forchuk, C., Martin, M.-L., Chan, L., & Jensen, E. (2005). Therapeutic relationships: From psychiatric hospital to community. *Journal of Psychiatric and Mental Health Nursing, 12*(5), 556–564. https://doi.org/10.1111/j.1365-2850.2005.00873.x

Forchuk, C., Martin, M.-L., Corring, D., Sherman, D., Srivastava, R., Harerimana, B., & Cheng, R. (2019). Cost-effectiveness of the implementation of a transitional discharge model for community integration of psychiatric clients: Practice insights and policy implications. *International Journal of Mental Health, 48*(3), 236–249. https://doi.org/10.1080/00207411.2019.1649237

Forchuk, C., Martin, M.-L., Jensen, E., Ouseley, S., Sealy, P., Beal, G., Reynolds, W., & Sharkey, S. (2012). Integrating the transitional relationship model into clinical practice. *Archives of Psychiatric Nursing, 26*(5), 374–381. https://doi.org/10.1016/j.apnu.2011.12.002

Forchuk, C., Martin, M.-L., Jensen, E., Ouseley, S., Sealy, P., Beal, G., Reynolds, W., & Sharkey, S. (2013). Integrating an evidence-based intervention into clinical practice: "Transitional relationship model". *Journal of Psychiatric and Mental Health Nursing, 20*(7), 584–594. https://doi.org/10.1111/j.1365-2850.2012.01956.x

Forchuk, C., Martin, M.-L., Sherman, D., Corring, D., Srivastava, R., O-Regan, T., Gyamifi, S., & Harerimana, B. (2020). An ethnographic study of the implementation of a transitional discharge model: Peer supporters' perspectives. *International Journal of Mental Health Systems, 14*(18), 1–11. https://doi.org/10.1186/s13033-020-00353-y

Forchuk, C., Martin, M.-L., Sherman, D., Corring, D., Srivastava, R., O'Regan, T., Gyamifi, S., & Harerimana, B . (2019). Healthcare professionals' perceptions of the implementation of the transitional discharge model for community integration of psychiatric clients. *International Journal of Mental Health Nursing, 29*(3), 498–507. https://doi.org/10.1111/inm.12687

Forchuk, C., & Reynolds, W. (2001). Clients' reflections on relationships with nurses: Comparisons from Canada and Scotland. *Journal of Psychiatric & Mental Health Nursing, 8*(1), 357–364. https://doi.org /10.1046/j.1365-2850.2001.00344.x

Forchuk, C., Reynolds, W., Sharkey, S., Martin, M. L., & Jensen, E. (2007a). The transitional discharge model: Comparing implementation in Canada and Scotland. *Journal of Psychosocial Nursing and Mental Health Services, 45*(11), 31–38. https://doi.org/10.3928/02793695-20071101-07

Forchuk, C., Reynolds, W., Sharkey, S., Martin, M. L., & Jensen, E. (2007b). Transitional discharge based on therapeutic relationships: State of the art. *Archives of Psychiatric Nursing, 21*(2), 80–86. https://do i.org/10.1016/j.apnu.2006.11.002

Forchuk, C., Schofield, R., Martin, M. L., Sircelj, M., Woodcox, V., Jewell, J., Valledov, T., Overby, B., & Chan, L. (1998). Bridging the discharge process: Staff and client experiences over time. *Journal of the American Psychiatric Nurses Association, 4*(4), 128–133. https://doi.org/10.1016/S1078-3903(98)90003-9

Forchuk, C., Solomon, M., & Virani, T. (2016). Peer support: An important part of transitional discharge. *Healthcare Quarterly (Toronto, Ontario), 18*(special issue), 32–36. https://doi.org/10.12927/hcq.2016 .24480

Forchuk, C., & Voorberg, N. (1991). Evaluating a community mental health program. *Canadian Journal of Nursing Administration, 4*(2), 16–20.

Forchuk, C., Westwell, J., Martin, M.-L., Bamber-Azzapardi, W., Kosterewa-Tolman, D., & Hux, M. (1998). Factors influencing movement of chronic psychiatric patients from the orientation to the working phase of the nurse-client relationship on an inpatient unit. *Perspectives in Psychiatric Care, 34*(1), 36–44. https://doi.org/10.1111/j.1744-6163.1998.tb00998.x

Forchuk, C., Westwell, J., Martin, M.-L., Bamber-Azzapardi, W., Kosterewa-Tolman, D., & Hux, M. (2000). The developing nurse-client relationship: Nurses' perspectives. *Journal of the American Psychiatric Nurses Association, 6*(1), 3–10. Copyright© (SAGE Publications). https://doi.org/10.1177 %2F107839030000600102

Frank, A. F., & Gunderson, J. G. (1990). The role of the therapeutic alliance in the treatment of schizophrenia: Relationship to course and outcome. *Archives of General Psychiatry, 47*(3), 228–236. http://doi.org/10.1001/archpsyc.1990.01810150028006

Garfinkel, P. E., Dorian, B., Sadavoy, J., & Bagby, R. M. (1997). Boundary violations and departments of psychiatry. *Canadian Journal of Psychiatry, 42*(7), 764–770. https://doi.org/10.1177%2F070674379 704200710

Gates, L. B., & Akabas, S. H. (2007). Developing strategies to integrate peer providers into the staff of mental health agencies. *Administration and Policy in Mental Health and Mental Health Services Research, 34*(3), 293–306. https://doi.org/10.1007/s10488-006-0109-4

Gilbert, P. (Ed.). (2005). *Compassion: Conceptualizations, research and use in psychotherapy.* Routledge.

Gilbert, P. (Ed.). (2017). *Compassion: Concepts, research and applications.* Taylor & Francis.

Gilbert, P., & Mascaro, J. (2017). Compassion: Fears, blocks, and resistances: An evolutionary investigation. In E. M. Seppala, E. Simon-Thomas, S. L. Brown, M. C. Worline, C. D. Cameron, & J. R. Doty (Eds.), *The Oxford handbook of compassion and science* (pp. 41–49). Oxford University Press.

Gladstein, G. (1977). Empathy and counselling outcome: An empirical and conceptual review. *Counseling Psychologist, 6*, 70–79. https://doi.org/10.1177%2F001100007700600427

Glembocki, M. M., & Fitzpatrick, J. (2013). *Advancing professional nursing practice: Relationship-based care and the ANA standards of professional nursing practice.* Creative Health Care Management.

Goetz, J. L., Keltner, D., & Simon-Thomas, E. (2010). Compassion. An evolutionary analysis and empirical review. *Psychological Bulletin, 136*(3), 351–374. https://doi.org/10.1037/a0018807

Gosselin, E., Paul-Savoie, E., Lavoie, S., & Bourgault, P. (2015). Validity of the French version of the Reynolds empathy scale among intensive care nurses. *Journal of Nursing Measurements, 23*(1), E16–26. https://doi.org/10.1891/1061-3749.23.1.E16

Graneheim, U. H., & Lundman, B. (2004). Qualitative content analysis in nursing research: Concepts, procedures and measures to achieve trustworthiness. *Nurse Education Today*, *24*(2), 105–112. https://doi.org/10.1016/j.nedt.2003.10.001

Greenberg, G., & Rosenheck, R. (2005). Special section on the GAF: Continuity of care and clinical outcomes in a national health system. *Psychiatric Services*, *56*(4), 427–433. https://doi.org/10.1176/appi.ps.56.4.427

Gregg, D. (1954). The psychiatric nurse's role. *American Journal of Nursing*, *54*(7), 848–851.

Guldager, R., Willis, K., Larsen, K., & Poulsen, I. (2019). Nurses' contribution to relatives' involvement in neurorehabilitation: Facilitators and barriers. *Nursing Open*, *6*(4), 1314–1322. https://doi.org/10.1002/nop2.326

Gutheil, T. G., & Gabbard, G. O. (1993). The concept of boundaries in clinical practice: Theoretical and risk-management dimensions. *American Journal of Psychiatry*, *150*(2), 188–196. https://doi.org/10.1176/ajp.150.2.188

Gutheil, T. G., & Simon, R. I. (1995). Between the chair and the door: Boundary issues in the therapeutic "transition zone". *Harvard Review of Psychiatry*, *2*(6), 336–340. https://doi.org/10.3109/10673229509017154

Gutheil, T. G., & Simon, R. I. (2002). Non-sexual boundary crossings and boundary violations: The ethical dimension. *Psychiatric Clinics of North America*, *25*(3), 585–592. https://doi.org/10.1016/S0193-953X(01)00012-0

Gyamfi, S. K. (2016). *Comprehensive psychiatry for nurses*. Beap Publications.

Halter, M. J. (Ed.). (2014). *Varcarolis' foundations of psychiatric mental health nursing: A clinical approach* (7th ed.). Elsevier Saunders.

Hansson, L., Jormfeldt, H., Svedberg, P., & Svensson, B. (2013). Mental health professionals' attitudes towards people with mental illness: Do they differ from attitudes held by people with mental illness? *International Journal of Social Psychiatry*, *59*(1), 48–54. https://doi.org/10.1177/0020764011423176

Happell, B., Waks, S. Bocking, J., Horgan, A., Manning, F., Greaney, S., Goodwin, J., Scholz, B., van der Vaart, K. J., Allon, J., Hals, E., Granerud, A., Doody, R., MacGabhann, L., Russell, S., Griffin, M., Lahti, M., Ellila, H., Pulli, J.,…Biering, P. (2019). "I felt some prejudice in the back of my head": Nursing students' perspectives on learning about mental health from "Experts by Experience". *Journal of Psychiatric and Mental Health Nursing*, *26*(7–8), 233–243. https://doi.org/10.1111/jpm.12540

Hardiman, E. R. (2004). Networks of caring: A qualitative study of social support in consumer-run mental health agencies. *Qualitative Social Work*, *3*(4), 431–448. https://doi.org/10.1177/1473325004048024

Hardy, C. (2017). Empathising with patients: The role of interaction and narrative in providing patient care. *Medicine, Health Care, and Philosophy*, *20*(2), 237–248. https://doi.org/10.1007/s11019-016-9746-x

Hartley, D., & Strupp, H. (1983). The therapeutic alliance relationship to outcome in brief psychotherapy. In J. Masling (Ed.), *Empirical studies of psychoanalytic theories* (Vol. 1., pp. 1–27). Analytic Press.

Haynes, N., & Strode, P. (2011). Opening doors to recovery: A novel community navigation service for people with serious mental illnesses. *Psychiatric Services*, *62*, 1270–1272. https://doi.org/10.1176/ps.62.11.pss6211_1270

Heifner, C. (1997). The male experience of depression. *Perspectives in Psychiatric Care*, *33*(2), 10–18. https://doi.org/10.1111/j.1744-6163.1997.tb00536.x

Hengartner, M., Loch, A., Lawson, F., Guarniero, F., Wang, Y.-P., Rössler, W., & Gattaz, W. (2013). Public stigmatization of different mental disorders: A comprehensive attitude survey. *Epidemiology and Psychiatric Sciences*, *22*(3), 269–274. https://doi.org/10.1017/S2045796012000376

Henry, B. W., Block, D. E., Ciesla, J. R., McGowan, B. A., & Vozenilek, J. A. (2017). Clinician behaviors in telehealth care delivery: A systematic review. *Advances in Health Sciences Education*, *22*(4), 869–888. https://doi.org/10.1007/s10459-016-9717-2

Hills, M. D., & Knowles, D. (1983). Nurses' levels of empathy and respect in simulated interaction with patients. *International Journal of Nursing Studies*, *20*(2), 83–87. https://doi.org/10.1016/0020-7489(83)90003-2

Hirschmann, M. J. (1989). Psychiatric and mental health nurses' beliefs about therapeutic paradox. *Journal of Child Psychiatric Nursing*, *2*(1), 7–13. https://doi.org/10.1111/j.1744-6171.1989.tb00355.x

Ho, A., & Quick, O. (2018). Leaving patients to their own devices? Smart technology, safety and therapeutic relationships. *BMC Medical Ethics, 19*(18), 1–6. https://doi.org/10.1186/s12910-018-0255-8

Hodges, J. Q., Markward, M., Keele, C., & Evans, C. J. (2003). Use of self-help services and consumer satisfaction with professional mental health services. *Psychiatric Services, 54*(8), 1161–1163. https://doi.org/10.1176/appi.ps.54.8.1161

Holbert, S., Martin, M.-L., Lysiak-Globe, T., Forchuk, C., Jensen, E., Coatsworth-Pusposky, R., & Ricci, A. (2003, March 27–29). *Staff education to support research* [Paper presentation]. NACNS National Conference: CNS Excellence in Clinical Practice and Leadership: Many Faces; One Mission, Pittsburgh, PA.

Holden, G. W., & Smith, M. M. (2018). Attitudes. In M. H. Bornstein (Ed.), *The SAGE encyclopedia of lifespan human development* (pp. 182–183). SAGE Publications Ltd.

Horowitz, L. (1974). *Clinical Prediction in Psychotherapy*. Aronson.

Horvath, A. O. (2001). The alliance. *Psychotherapy: Theory, Research, Practice, Training, 38*(4), 365–372. https://psycnet.apa.org/doi/10.1037/0033-3204.38.4.365

Horvath, A. O., & Greenberg, L. (1986). The development of the working alliance inventory. In L. Greenberg & W. Pinsof (Eds.), *The psychotherapeutic process: A research handbook* (pp. 529–556). Gulford Press.

Horvath, A. O., & Greenberg, L. (1989). Development and validation of the working alliance inventory. *Journal of Counseling Psychology, 36*(2), 223–233. https://doi.org/10.1037/0022-0167.36.2.223

Hutchison, P. J., McLaughlin, K., Corbridge, T., Michelson, K. N., Emanuel, L., Sporn, P. H., & Crowley-Matoka, M. (2016). Dimensions and role-specific mediators of surrogate trust in the ICU. *Critical Care Medicine, 44*(12), 2208–2214. https://doi.org/10.1097/ccm.0000000000001957

International Council of Nurses. (2012). *The ICN code of ethics for nurses.* Author. https://www.icn.ch/sites/default/files/inline-files/2012_ICN_Codeofethicsfornurses_%20eng.pdf

IQVIA Institute. (2017). *The growing value of digital health: Evidence and impact on human health and the healthcare system.* Institute report. https://www.iqvia.com/insights/the-iqvia-institute/reports/the-growing-value-of-digital-health

Islam, M. A., Siddique, M. N. H., & Karim, A. A. M. E. (1991). *Participatory action research.* Integrated Development Programme, BRAC.

Jacob, K. S. (2015). Recovery model of mental illness: A complementary approach to psychiatric care. *Indian Journal of Psychological Medicine, 37*(2), 117–119.

Jayaram, G. (2015). Handoffs in psychiatry. In G. Jayaram (Ed.), *Practicing patient safety in psychiatry* (pp. 29–45). Oxford University Press.

Jazaieri, H., Jinpa, G. T., McGonigal, K., Rosenberg, E. L., Finkelstein, J., Simon-Thomas, E., Cullen, M., Doty, J. R., Gross, J. J., & Goldin, P. R. (2013). Enhancing compassion: A randomized controlled trial of a compassion cultivation training program. *Journal of Happiness Studies, 14*(4), 1113–1126. https://doi.org/10.1007/s10902-012-9373-z

Jenkins-Guarnieri, M. A., Pruitt, L. D., Luxton, D. D., & Johnson, K. (2015). Patient perceptions of telemental health: Systematic review of direct comparisons to in-person psychotherapeutic treatments. *Telemedicine and e-Health, 21*(8), 652–660. https://doi.org/10.1089/tmj.2014.0165

Júnior, F., Marques, H., Desviat, M., & Silva, P. R. F. D. (2016). Psychiatric reform in Rio de Janeiro: The current situation and future perspectives. *Ciencia & Saude Coletiva, 21*(5), 1449–1460. http://dx.doi.org/10.1590/1413-81232015215.00872016

Kalkman, M. (1967). *Psychiatric nursing.* McGraw-Hill.

Kaplan, K., Salzer, M. S., & Brusilovskiy, E. (2012). Community participation as a predictor of recovery-oriented outcomes among emerging and mature adults with mental illnesses. *Psychiatric Rehabilitation Journal, 35*(3), 219–229. https://doi.org/10.2975/35.3.2012.219.229

Keltner, D., & Goetz, J. (2007). Compassion. In R. F. Baumeister & K. D. Vohs (Eds.), *Encyclopedia of social psychology* (pp. 160–161). SAGE Publications Ltd.

Kennedy, B. M., Rehman, M., Johnson, W. D., Magee, M. B., Leonard, R., & Katzmarzyk, P. T. (2017). Healthcare providers versus patients' understanding of health beliefs and values. *Patient Experience Journal, 4*(3), 29–37. https://doi.org/10.35680/2372-0247.1237

Kerse, N., Buetow, S., Mainous III, A. G., Young, G., Coster, G., & Arroll, B. (2004). Physician-patient relationship and medication compliance: A primary care investigation. *Annals of Family Medicine, 2*(5), 455–461. https://dx.doi.org/10.1370%2Fafm.139

Kitenge, C. (2017). *Nurses' attitudes towards HIV positive patients in Swaziland.* Unpublished master's dissertation. Swaziland Christian University.

Knapp, M., McDaid, D., & Mossialos, E. (2006). *Mental health policy and practice across Europe.* McGraw-Hill.

Knobloch-Fedders, L. (2008). The importance of the relationship with the therapist. *Clinical Science Insights: Knowledge Families Count On, 1,* 1–3.

Kornhaber, R., Walsh, K., Duff, J., & Walker, K. (2016). Enhancing adult therapeutic interpersonal relationships in the acute health care setting: An integrative review. *Journal of Multidisciplinary Healthcare, 6*(9), 537–546. https://dx.doi.org/10.2147%2FJMDH.S116957

Krupinski, J. (1995). De-institutionalization of psychiatric patients: Progress or abandonment? *Social Science & Medicine, 40*(5), 577–579. http://dx.doi.org/10.1016/0277-9536(95)80001-Z

Kutchins, H. (1991). The fiduciary relationship: The legal basis for social workers' responsibilities to clients. *Social Work, 36*(2), 106–113. https://doi.org/10.1093/sw/36.2.106

Lambert, M. J., & Barley, D. E. (2001). Research summary on the therapeutic relationship and psychotherapy outcome. *Psychotherapy: Theory, Research, Practice, Training, 38*(4), 357–361. https://psycnet.apa.org/doi/10.1037/0033-3204.38.4.357

La Monica, E. L., Wolf, R. M., Madea, A. R., & Oberst, M. T. (1987). Empathy and nursing care outcomes. *Scholarly Inquiry for Nursing Practice, 1*(3), 197–213.

Laroi, F., Luhrmann, T. M., Bell, V., Christian, W. A., Deshpande, S., Fernyhough, C., Jenkins, J., & Woods, A. (2014). Culture and hallucinations: Overview and future directions. *Schizophrenia Bulletin, 40*(4), S213–S220. https://doi.org/10.1093/schbul/sbu012

Leamy, M., Bird, V., Le Boutillier, C., Williams, J., & Slade, M. (2011). Conceptual framework for personal recovery in mental health: Systematic review and narrative synthesis. *British Journal of Psychiatry, 199*(6), 445–452. https://doi.org/10.1192/bjp.bp.110.083733

LeCompte, M. D., & Schensul, J. J. (1999). *Analyzing & interpreting ethnographic data* (Vol. 5). Rowman Altamira.

Ledoux, K., Forchuk, C., Higgins, C., & Rudnick, A. (2018). The effect of organizational and personal variables on the ability to practice compassionately. *Applied Nursing Research, 41,* 15–20. https://doi.org/10.1016/j.apnr.2018.03.001

Legg, M., Occhipinti, S., Youl, P., Dunn, J., & Chambers, S. K. (2017). Needy or resilient? How women with breast cancer think about peer support. *Psycho-Oncology, 26*(12), 2307–2310. https://doi.org/10.1002/pon.4401

Lehman, A. (1988). A quality of life interview for the chronically mentally ill. *Evaluation and Program Planning, 111*(1), 51–62. https://doi.org/10.1016/0149-7189(88)90033-X

Lehman, A., Kernan, E., & Postrado, L. (1995). *Toolkit evaluating quality of life for persons with severe mental illness.* Evaluation Centre and Human Services Research Institute. https://www.hsri.org/publication/toolkit_evaluating_quality_of_life_for_persons_with_severe_mental_illn

Leininger, M. M. (1985). Ethnography and ethnonnursing: Models and modes of qualitative data analysis. In M. M. Leininger (Ed.), *Qualitative research methods in nursing* (pp. 33–72). Grune & Stratton.

Lemmens, L., Galindo-Garre, F., Arntz, A., Peeters, F., Hollon, S., Deruibeis, R., & Huibers, M. (2017). Exploring mechanisms of change in cognitive therapy and interpersonal psychotherapy for adult depression. *Behaviour Research and Therapy, 94,* 81–82. https://doi.org/10.1016/j.brat.2017.05.005

Link, B. G., & Phelan, J. C. (2001). Conceptualizing stigma. *Annual Review of Sociology, 27,* 363–385. https://doi.org/10.1146/annurev.soc.27.1.363

Little, J., Hirdes, J. P., Perlman, C. M., & Meyer, S. B. (2019). Clinical predictors of delayed discharges in inpatient mental health settings across Ontario. *Administration and Policy in Mental Health and Mental Health Services Research, 46*(1), 105–114. https://doi.org/10.1007/s10488-018-0898-2

Loch, A. A. (2014). Discharged from a mental health admission ward: Is it safe to go home? A review on the negative outcomes of psychiatric hospitalization. *Psychology Research and Behaviour Management, 7,* 137. https://doi.org/10.2147/PRBM.S35061

Loch, A. A., Wang, Y.-P., Guarniero, F. B., Lawson, F. L., Hengartner, M. P., Rössler, W., & Gattaz, W. F. (2014). Patterns of stigma toward schizophrenia among the general population: A latent profile analysis. *International Journal of Social Psychiatry, 60*(6), 595–605. https://doi.org/10.1177/0020764013507248

Lown, B. A. (2015). Compassion is a necessity and an individual and collective responsibility: Comment on "Why and how is compassion necessary to provide good quality healthcare?". *International Journal of Health Policy Management, 4*(9), 613–614. https://doi.org/10.15171/ijhpm.2015.110

Lown, B. A., Muncer, S. J., & Chadwick, R. (2015). Can compassionate healthcare be measured? The Schwartz center compassionate care scale™. *Patient Education and Counseling, 98*(8), 1005–1010. https://doi.org/10.1016/j.pec.2015.03.019

Luberto, C. M., Shinday, N., Song, R., Philpotts, L. L., Park, E. R., Ficchione, G. L., & Yeh, G. Y. (2018). A systematic review and meta-analysis of the effects of meditation on empathy, compassion, and prosocial behaviors. *Mindfulness, 9*(3), 708–724. https://doi.org/10.1007/s12671-017-0841-8

Luborsky, L. (1976). Helping alliances in psychotherapy. In J. Claghom (Ed.), *Successful psychotherapy* (pp. 92–118). Brunner/Mazel.

MacKay, R. C., Hughes, J. R., & Carver, E. J. (Eds.). (1990). *Empathy in the helping relationship.* Springer.

Madi, N., Zhao, H., & Li, J. F. (2007). Hospital readmissions for patients with mental illness in Canada. *Healthcare Quarterly (Toronto, Ontario), 10*(2), 30–32.

Maio, G. R., & Haddock, G. (2010). The influence of attitudes on information processing and behavior. In G. R. Maio & G. Haddock (Eds.), *The psychology of attitudes and attitude change* (pp. 47–66). SAGE Publications Ltd.

Mancini, M. A. (2018). An exploration of factors that effect the implementation of peer support services in community mental health settings. *Community Mental Health Journal, 54*(2), 127–137. https://doi.org/10.1007/s10597-017-0145-4

Manfrida, G., Albertini, V., & Eisenberg, E. (2017). Connected: Recommendations and techniques in order to employ internet tools for the enhancement of online therapeutic relationships. Experiences from Italy. *Contemporary Family Therapy, 39*(4), 314–328. https://doi.org/10.1007/s10591-017-9439-5

Manfrin-Ledet, L., Porche, D. J., & Eymard, A. S. (2015). Professional boundary violations: A literature review. *Home Healthcare Now, 33*(6), 326–332. https://doi.org/10.1097/nhh.0000000000000249

Mannion, R. (2014). Enabling compassionate healthcare: Perils, prospects and perspectives. *International Journal of Health Policy Management, 2*(3), 115–117. https://dx.doi.org/10.15171%2Fijhpm.2014.34

Manthey, M. (2015). *Primary nursing: Person-centered care delivery system design.* Springer.

Martin, M.-L. (2014). Transitions. In C. Webster, Q. Haque, & S. Hucker (Eds.), *Violence risk, assessment and management* (2nd ed., pp. 98–105). John Wiley.

Martin, M.-L., Forchuk, C., Coatsworth-Puspoky, R., Lysiak-Globe, T., Ricci, A., Jensen, E., Sloan, K., & Holbert, S. (2002, May 15). *Staff education to support research. Therapeutic relationships: From hospital to community.* Dissemination Conference. London.

Martin, M.-L., Jensen, E., Coatsworth-Puspoky, R., Forchuk, C., Lysiak-Globe, T., & Beal, G. (2007). Integrating an evidenced-based research intervention in the discharge of mental health clients. *Archives of Psychiatric Nursing, 21*(2), P101–111. https://doi.org/10.1016/j.apnu.2006.11.004

Martin, M.-L., & Kirkpatrick, H. (1987). *Nursing theories used by staff nurses.* Unpublished manuscript. Hamilton Psychiatric Hospital.

Martin, M.-L., & Kirkpatrick, H. (1989). *Nursing theories used by staff nurses: A two year re-evaluation.* Unpublished manuscript. Hamilton Psychiatric Hospital.

Marwick, A. E., & Boyd, D. (2010). I tweet honestly, I tweet passionately: Twitter users, context collapse, and the imagined audience. *New Media and Society, 13*(1), 114–133. https://doi.org/10.1177%2F1461444810365313

May, R. (1950). *The meaning of anxiety.* Ronald Press Co.

McGinnis, J. M., Stuckhardt, L., Saunders, R., & Smith, M. (Eds.). (2013). *Best care at lower cost: The path to continuously learning health care in America.* National Academies Press.

McGonigal, K. (2017, July 5). How to overcome stress by seeing other people's joy. *Greater Good Magazine.* https://greatergood.berkeley.edu/article/item/how:to_overcome_stress_by_seeing_other_peoples_joy

McQueen, A. (2000). Nurse-patient relationship and partnership in hospital care. *Journal of Clinical Nursing*, *9*(5), 723–731. https://doi.org/10.1046/j.1365-2702.2000.00424.x

Mead, G. H. (1934). *Mind, self, and society*. University of Chicago Press.

Mental Health Commission of Canada. (2013). *Opening minds programs*. https://www.mentalhealthcommission.ca/sites/default/files/Stigma_OM_Programs_Listed_by_Province_ENG_0.pdf

Mental Health Commission of Canada. (2014). *E-Mental health in Canada: Transforming the mental health system using technology*. https://www.mentalhealthcommission.ca/sites/default/files/MHCC_E-Mental_Health-Briefing_Document_ENG_0.pdf

Mental Health Commission of Canada. (2015). *Guidelines for recovery-oriented practice: Hope. Dignity. Inclusion*. Author.

Mercer, S., & Reynolds, W. (2002). Empathy and quality of care. *British Journal of General Practice*, *52*(Supplement), S9–S12.

Mereness, D. (1966). *Psychiatric nursing: Developing psychiatric nursing skills* (Vols. 1–2). Wm. C. Brown.

Merriam-Webster. (n.d.a.) *Assumption*. https://www.merriamwebster.com/dictionary/assumption

Merriam-Webster. (n.d.b.). *Belief*. https://www.merriam-webster.com/dictionary/belief

Miller, N. E., & Dollard, J. (1941). *Social learning and imitation*. Yale University Press.

Min, S.-Y., Whitecraft, J., Rothbard, A. B., & Salzer, M. S. (2007). Peer support for persons with co-occurring disorders and community tenure: A survival analysis. *Psychiatric Rehabilitation Journal*, *30*(3), 207–213. https://doi.org/10.2975/30.3.2007.207.213

Mings, E., & Cramp, J. (2014). *Best practices in peer support: 2014 final report*. http://eenet.ca/wp-content/uploads/2014/08/Best-Practices-PeerSupport-Final-Report-2014.pdf

Miserandino, M. (2007). Attitude formation. In R. F. Baumeister & K. D. Vohs (Eds.), *Encyclopedia of social psychology* (pp. 66–67). SAGE Publications Ltd.

Moll, S., Holmes, J., Geronimo, J., & Sherman, D. (2009). Work transitions for peer support providers in traditional mental health programs: Unique challenges and opportunities. *Work*, *33*(4), 449–458. https://doi.org/10.3233/WOR-2009-0893

Moore, C., Wisnivesky, J., Williams, S., & McGinn, T. (2003). Medical errors related to discontinuity of care from an inpatient to an outpatient setting. *Journal of General Internal Medicine*, *18*(8), 646–651. https://doi.org/10.1046/j.1525-1497.2003.20722.x

Moreno-Poyato, A. R., Delgado-Hito, P., Sarez-Perez, R., Lluch Canut, M., Merino, R., Francisco, J., & Monteso Curto, P. (2018). Improving the therapeutic relationship in inpatient psychiatric care: Assessment of the therapeutic alliance and empathy after implementing evidence-based practices resulting from participatory action research. *Perspectives in Psychiatric Care*, *54*(2), 300–308. https://doi.org/10.1111/ppc.12238

Moreno-Poyato, A. R., Monteso-Curto, P., Delgado-Hilton, P., Suárez-Pérez, R., Aceña Domínguez, R., Carreras-Salvador, R., Leyva-Moral, J. M., Lluch-Canut, T., & Roldán-Merino, J. F. (2016). The therapeutic relationship in inpatient psychiatric care: A narrative review of the perspective of nurses and patients. *Archives of Psychiatric Nursing*, *30*(6), 782–787. http://doi.org/10.1016/j.apnu.2016.03.001

Morris, M. E., & Aguilera, A. (2012). Mobile, social, and wearable computing and the evolution of psychological practice. *Professional Psychology: Research and Practice*, *43*(6), 622–626. https://doi.org/10.1037/a0029041

Morse, J., Anderson, G., Bottor, J., Yonge, O., & Solberg, S. (1992). Exploring empathy: A conceptual fit for nursing practice? *Image - the Journal of Nursing Scholarship*, *24*(4), 273–280. https://doi.org/10.1111/j.1547-5069.1992.tb00733.x

Murphy, H., Tubritt, J., & O'Higgins Norman, J. (2018). The role of empathy in preparing teachers to tackle bullying. *Journal of New Approaches in Educational Research*, *7*(1), 17–22. https://doi.org/10.7821/naer.2018.1.261

Murray, B., & McCrone, S. (2015). An integrative review of promoting trust in the patient primary care provider relationship. *Journal of Advanced Nursing*, *71*(1), 3–23. https://doi.org/10.1111/jan.12502

Nakash, O., Cohen, M., & Nagar, M. (2018). "How should I do it"? Clinical dilemmas therapists struggle with during the mental health intake. *Qualitative Social Work*, *18*(4), 655–676. https://doi.org/10.1177/%2F1473325018755889

Naylor, M., Brooten, D., Jones, R., Lavizzo-Mourey, R., Mezey, M., & Pauly, M. (1994). Comprehensive discharge planning for the hospitalized elderly. A randomized clinical trial. *Annals of Internal Medicine*, 120(12), 999–1006. https://doi.org/10.7326/0003-4819-120-12-199406150-00005

Neff, K. D. (2003). The development and validation of a scale to measure self-compassion. *Self and Identity*, 2(3), 223–250. https://psycnet.apa.org/doi/10.1080/15298860309027

NHS Commissioning Board. (2012). *Compassion in practice: Nursing, midwifery and care staff: Our vision and strategy*. https://www.england.nhs.uk/wp-content/uploads/2012/12/compassion-in-practice.pdf

Niimura, J., Tanoue, M., & Nakanishi, M. (2016). Challenges following discharge from acute psychiatric inpatient care in Japan: Patients' perspectives. *Journal of Psychiatric and Mental Health Nursing*, 23(9–10), 576–584. https://doi.org/10.1111/jpm.12341

Norcross, J. C., & Lambert, M. J. (2018). Psychotherapy relationships that work III. *Psychotherapy*, 55(4), 303–315. https://doi.org/10.1037/pst0000193

Norcross, J. C., & Wampold, B. E. (2011). Evidence-based therapy relationships: Research conclusions and clinical practices. *Psychotherapy*, 48(1), 98–102. https://doi.org/10.1037/a0022161

Nurses' Association of New Brunswick. (2015). *Standards for the therapeutic nurse-client relationship*. Author. http://www.nanb.nb.ca/media/resource/NANB-StandardsNurseClientRelation-E-2015-10.pdf

Nyblade, L., Stockton, M. A., Giger, K., Bond, V., Ekstrand, M. L., Mc Lean, R., Mitchelle,E. M. H., Nelson, L. R. E., Sapag, J. C., Siraprapasiri, T., Turan, J., & Wouters, E. (2019). Stigma in health facilities: Why it matters and how we can change it. *BMC Medicine*, 17(25). https://doi.org/10.1186/s12916-019-1256-2

O'Brien, A. J. (2001). The therapeutic relationship: Historical development and contemporary significance. *Journal of Psychiatric and Mental Health Nursing*, 82(2), 129–137. https://doi.org/10.1046/j.1365-2850.2001.00367.x

Ochocka, J., Nelson, G., Janzen, R., & Trainor, J. (2006). A longitudinal study of mental health consumer/survivor initiatives: Part 3 - A qualitative study of impacts of participation on new members. *Journal of Community Psychology*, 34(3), 273–283. https://doi.org/10.1002/jcop.20099

Office of the Auditor General of Ontario. (2016). *Annual report 2016* (Vol. 1). https://www.auditor.on.ca/en/content/annualreports/arreports/en16/2016AR_v1_en_web.pdf

Olfson, M., Mechanic, D., Boyer, C. A., & Hansell, S. (1998). Linking inpatients with schizophrenia to outpatient care. *Psychiatric Services (Washington, D.C.)*, 49(7), 911–917. https://doi.org/10.1176/ps.49.7.911

Olfson, M., Mechanic, D., Hansell, S., Boyer, C. A., Walkup, J., & Weiden, P. J. (2000). Predicting medication noncompliance after hospital discharge among patients with schizophrenia. *Psychiatric Services*, 51(2), 216–222. https://doi.org/10.1176/appi.ps.51.2.216

Olson, R. P. (2006). *Mental health systems compared: Great Britain, Norway, Canada, and the United States*. Charles C Thomas Publisher.

Orlinsky, D. E., & Howard, K. I. (1978). The relation of process to outcome in psychotherapy. In S. L. Garfield & A. E. Bergin (Eds.), *Handbook of psychotherapy and behavior change* (pp. 311–381). John Wiley.

Osgood, C. E., Suci, G. J., & Tannenbaum, P. H. (1957). *Measurement of meaning*. University of Illinois Press.

Patterson, C. (1974). *Relationship counselling and psychotherapy*. Harper and Row.

Paul, M., O'Hara, L., Tah, P., Street, C., Mara, A., Purper Ouakil, D., Santosh, P., Signorini, G., Singh, S. P., Tuomainen, H., McNicholas, F., & MILESTONE Consortium. (2018). A systematic review of the literature on ethical aspects of transitional care between child- and adult-orientated health services. *BMC Medical Ethics*, 19(73). https://doi.org/10.1186/s12910-018-0276-3

Pazargadi, M., Moghadam, M. F., Khoshknab, M. F., Renani, H. A., & Molazem, Z. (2015). The therapeutic relationship in the shadow: Nurses' experiences of barriers to the nurse-patient relationship in the psychiatric ward. *Issues in Mental Health Nursing*, 36(7), 551–557. https://doi.org/10.3109/01612840.2015.1014585

Pedersen, P. B., & Kolstad, A. (2009). De-institutionalisation and trans-institutionalisation - Changing trends of inpatient care in Norwegian mental health institutions 1950–2007. *International Journal of Mental Health Systems*, 3(28). https://dx.doi.org/10.1186%2F1752-4458-3-28

Peplau, H. E. (1952). *Interpersonal relations in nursing*. G. P. Putnam's Sons.

Peplau, H. E. (1962). Interpersonal techniques: The crux of psychiatric nursing. *American Journal of Nursing, 62*, 50–54. https://doi.org/10.1007/978-1-349-13441-0_13

Peplau, H. E. (1964). *Basic principles of patient counselling.* Smith, Kline and French Laboratories.

Peplau, H. E. (1965). The heart of nursing: Interpersonal relations. *Canadian Nurse, 61*(4), 273–275.

Peplau, H. E. (1971). Process and concept of learning. In S. F. Burd & M. A. Marshall (Eds.), *Some clinical approaches to psychiatric nursing* (pp. 333–336). MacMillan.

Peplau, H. E. (1973a). *The concept of psychotherapy* [Audio tape]. PSF Productions.

Peplau, H. E. (1973b). *The orientation phase* [Audio tape]. PSF Productions.

Peplau, H. E. (1973c). *The working phase* [Audio tape]. PSF Productions.

Peplau, H. E. (1973d). *The resolution phase* [Audio tape]. PSF Productions.

Peplau, H. E. (1987). Nursing science: A historical perspective. In R. Parse (Ed.), *Nursing science: Major paradigms, theories, and critiques* (pp. 13–30). W. B. Saunders Co.

Peplau, H. E. (1988a). *Interpersonal relations in nursing.* MacMillan (Original work published 1952, New York: G. P. Putnam's Sons).

Peplau, H. E. (1988b). *Substance and scope of psychiatric nursing* [Oral paper]. Canadian Conference on Psychiatric Nursing, Montreal, QC.

Peplau, H. E. (1989a). Anxiety, self and hallucinations. In A. W. O'Toole & S. R. Welt (Eds.), *Interpersonal theory in nursing practice: Selected works of Hildegard E. Peplau* (pp. 270–326). Springer.

Peplau, H. E. (1989b). Theory: The professional dimension. In A. W. O'Toole & S. R. Welt (Eds.), *Interpersonal theory in nursing practice: Selected works of Hildegard E. Peplau* (pp. 21–41). Springer.

Peplau, H. E. (1989c). Investigative counseling. In A. W. O'Toole & S. R. Welt (Eds.), *Interpersonal theory in nursing practice: Selected works of Hildegard E. Peplau* (pp. 205–229). Springer. Copyright 1986 by Schlesinger Library.

Peplau, H. E. (1989d). Therapeutic nurse-patient interaction. In A. W. O'Toole & S. R. Welt (Eds.), *Interpersonal theory in nursing practice: Selected works of Hildegard E. Peplau.* (pp. 192–204). Springer.

Peplau, H. E. (1990). Interpersonal relations model: Theoretical constructs, principles and general applications. In W. Reynolds & D. Cormack (Eds.), *Psychiatric and mental health nursing: Theory and applications* (pp. 87–132). Chapman and Hall.

Peplau, H. E. (1991). *Interpersonal relations in nursing.* Springer. (Original work published 1952, New York: G. P. Putnam's Sons).

Peplau, H. E. (1996). The client diagnosed as schizophrenic. In S. Lego (Ed.), *Psychiatric nursing: A comprehensive reference* (pp. 291–295). Lippincott Williams & Wilkins.

Peplau, H. E. (1997). Peplau's theory of interpersonal relations. *Nursing Science Quarterly, 10*(4), 162–167. https://doi.org/10.1177%2F089431849701000407

Peternelj-Taylor, C. A., & Yonge, O. (2003). Exploring boundaries in the nurse-client relationship: Professional roles and responsibilities. *Perspectives in Psychiatric Care, 39*(2), 55–66. https://doi.org/10.1111/j.1744-6163.2003.tb00677.x

Poghosyan, L., Norful, A. A., Ghaffari, A., George, M., Chhabra, S., & Olfson, M. (2019). Mental health delivery in primary care: The perspectives of primary care providers. *Archives of Psychiatric Nursing, 33*(5), 63–67. https://doi.org/10.1016/j.apnu.2019.08.001

Portman, J. (2014). Morality and schadenfreude. In W. W. van Dijk & J. W. Ouwerkerk (Eds.), *Schadenfreude: Understanding pleasure at the misfortune of others* (pp. 17–28). Cambridge University Press.

Priebe, S., Badesconyi, A., Fioritti, A., Hansson, L., Kilian, R., Torres-Gonzales, F., Turner, T., & Wiersma, D. (2005). Reinstitutionalisation in mental health care: Comparison of data on service provision from six European countries. *BMJ, 330*(7483), 123–126. https://doi.org/10.1136/bmj.38296.611215.AE

Quackenbush, D. M., & Krasner, A. (2012). Avatar therapy: Where technology, symbols, culture, and connection collide. *Journal of Psychiatric Practice, 18*(6), 451–459. https://doi.org/10.1097/01.pra.0000422745.17990.be

Reamer, F. G. (2003). Boundary issues in social work: Managing dual relationships. *Social Work, 48*(1), 121–133. https://doi.org/10.1093/sw/48.1.121

Reamer, F. G. (2015). Clinical social work in a digital environment: Ethical and risk-management challenges. *Clinical Social Work Journal, 43*(2), 120–132. https://doi.org/10.1007/s10615-014-0495-0

Registered Nurses' Association of Ontario (RNAO). (2002/2006). *Establishing therapeutic relationships.* Author. https://rnao.ca/bpg/guidelines/establishing-therapeutic-relationships

Registered Nurses' Association of Ontario (RNAO). (2017). *RNAO nurse educator mental health and addiction resource.* Author. https://rnao.ca/bpg/initiatives/mhai/mhar

Reynolds, W. (1987). Empathy: We know what we mean, but what do we teach? *Nurse Education Today, 7*(6), 265–269. https://doi.org/10.1016/0260-6917(87)90127-4

Reynolds, W. J. (2000). *The measurement and development of empathy in nursing.* Ashgate Publishing Ltd.

Reynolds, W. (2006). 30th anniversary commentary on Morse, M; Bottoff, J., Anderson, G., Obrien, B. & Soldberg, S. (1992). Beyond empathy: Expanding expressions of caring. *Journal of Advanced Nursing, 17*, 809–821. In Journal of Advance Nursing, 30th Anniversary Issue, 88–89.

Reynolds, W. (2009). Developing empathy. In P. Barker (Ed.), *Psychiatric and mental health nursing: The craft of caring* (2nd ed., pp. 321–329). Arnold.

Reynolds, W. J., Lauder, W., Sharkey, S., Maciver, S., Veitch, T., & Cameron, D. (2004). The effects of a transitional discharge model for psychiatric patients. *Journal of Psychiatric and Mental Health Nursing, 11*(1), 82–88. https://doi.org/10.1111/j.1365-2850.2004.00692.x

Reynolds, W. J., & Scott, B. (2000). Do nurses and other professional helpers normally display much empathy? *Journal of Advanced Nursing, 31*(1), 226–234. https://doi.org/10.1046/j.1365-2648.2000.01242.x

Richards, P., Simpson, S., Bastiampillai, T., Pietrabissa, G., & Castelnuovo, G. (2018). The impact of technology on therapeutic alliance and engagement in psychotherapy: The therapist's perspective. *Clinical Psychologist, 22*(2), 171–181. https://doi.org/10.1111/cp.12102

Ridling, D. A., Lewis-Newby, M., & Lindsey, D. (2011). Family-centered care in the pediatric intensive care unit. In B. Fuhrman & J. Zimmerman (Eds.), *Pediatric critical care* (4th ed., pp. 92–101). Mosby.

Rivera, J. J., Sullivan, A. M., & Valenti, S. S. (2007). Adding consumer-providers to intensive case management: Does it improve outcome? *Psychiatric Services, 58*(6), 802–809. https://doi.org/10.1176/ps.2007.58.6.802

Roberts, L. W., & Torous, J. (2017). Preparing residents and fellows to address ethical issues in the use of mobile technologies in clinical psychiatry. *Academic Psychiatry, 41*(1), 132–134. https://doi.org/10.1007/s40596-016-0594-z

Rogers, C. (1957). The necessary and sufficient conditions of therapeutic personality change. *Journal of Consulting Psychology, 21*, 95–103. https://psycnet.apa.org/doi/10.1037/h0045357

Rogers, C. (1961). *On becoming a person.* Houghlin Mifflin.

Rogers, C. (1975). Empathic: An unappreciated way of being. *Counseling Psychologist, 5*, 2–10. https://doi.org/10.1177%2F001100007500500202

Rogers, C., & Truax, C. (1967). Conditions antecedent to change: A theoretical view. In C. R. Rogers (Ed.), *The therapeutic relationship and its impact: A study of psychotherapy with schizophrenics.* University of Wisconsin Press.

Rudnick, A. (2001). A meta-ethical critique of care ethics. *Theoretical Medicine and Bioethics, 22*(6), 505–517. https://doi.org/10.1023/A:1014485908290

Rudnick, A. (2002). The ground of dialogical bioethics. *Health Care Analysis, 10*(4), 391–402. https://doi.org/10.1023/A:1023431310918

Rudnick, A. (2019). Moral responsibility reconsidered: Integrating chance, choice and constraint. *International Journal of Philosophy, 7*(2), 48–54. https://doi.org/10.11648/j.ijp.20190702.11

Salyers, M. P., Hicks, L. J., McGuire, A. B., Baumgardner, H., Ring, K., & Kim, H.-W. (2009). A pilot to enhance the recovery orientation of assertive community treatment through peer-provided illness management and recovery. *American Journal of Psychiatric Rehabilitation, 12*(3), 191–204. https://doi.org/10.1080/15487760903066305

Scanlon, A. (2006). Psychiatric nurses' perceptions of the constituents of the therapeutic relationship: A grounded theory study. *Journal of Psychiatric and Mental Health Nursing, 13*(3), 319–329. https://doi.org/10.1111/j.1365-2850.2006.00958.x

Schofield, R., Valledor, T., Sircelj, M., Forchuk, C., Jewell, J., & Woodcox, V. (1997). Evaluation of bridging institution and housing - A joint consumer-care provider initiative. *Journal of Psychosocial Nursing and Mental Health Services, 35*(10), 9–14.

Schottenfeld, L., Petersen, D., Peikes, D., Ricciardi, R., Burak, H., McNellis, R., & Genevro, J. (2016). *Creating patient-centered team-based primary care* (AHRQ Pub. No. 16-0002-EF). Agency for Healthcare Research and Quality, Rockville, 1–27.

Schuster, R., Berger, T., & Laireiter, A. R. (2018). Computer and psychotherapy - Do they fit? Review of the state of development of internet-based and blended interventions in psychotherapy. *Psychotherapeut, 63*(4), 271–282. https://doi.org/10.1007/s00278-017-0214-8

Shea, S., & Lionis, C. (2017). The call for compassion in health care. In E. M. Seppala, E. Simon-Thomas, S. L. Brown, M. C. Worline, C. D. Cameron, & J. R. Doty (Eds.). *The Oxford handbook of compassion science* (pp. 457–485). Oxford University Press.

Shea, S., Wynyard, R., & Lionis, C. (Eds.). (2014). *Providing compassionate healthcare: Challenges in policy and practice.* Routledge.

Sibeoni, J., Verneuil, L., Poulmarc'h, L., Orri, M., Jean, E., Podlipski, M. A., Gerardin, P., & Revah-Levy, A. (2020). Obstacles and facilitators of therapeutic alliance among adolescents with anorexia nervosa, their parents and their psychiatrists: A qualitative study. *Clinical Child Psychology and Psychiatry, 25*(1), 16–32. https://doi.org./10.1177/1359104519882765

Sills, G. M. (1978). Hildegard E. Peplau: Leader, practitioner, academician, scholar and theorist. *Perspectives in Psychiatric Care, 16*(3), 122–128. https://doi.org/10.1111/j.1744-6163.1978.tb00928.x

Silva, M. C. (1986). Research testing nursing theory state of art. *Advances in Nursing Science, 9*(1), 1–11. https://doi.org/10.1097/00012272-198610000-00003

Simpson, E. L., & House, A. O. (2002). Involving users in the delivery and evaluation of mental health services: Systematic review. *BMJ (Clinical Research Ed).), 325*(1265). https://doi.org/10.1136/bmj.325.7375.1265

Sinclair, S., McClement, S., Raffin-Bouchal, S., Hack, T. F., Hagen, N. A., McConnell, S., & Chochinov, H. M. (2016). Compassion in health care: An empirical model. *Journal of Pain and Symptom Management, 51*(2), 193–203. https://doi.org/10.1016/j.jpainsymman.2015.10.009

Singer, T., & Klimecki, O. M. (2014). Empathy and compassion. *Current Biology, 24*(18), R875–R878. https://doi.org/10.1016/j.cub.2014.06.054

Slade, M. (2017). Implementing shared decision making in routine mental health care. *World Psychiatry, 16*(2), 146–153. https://doi.org/10.1002/wps.20412

Sloane, J. A. (1993). Offenses and defences against patients: A psychoanalytic view of the borderline between empathic failure and malpractice. *Canadian Journal of Psychiatry, 38*(4), 265–273. https://doi.org/10.1177/070674379303800408

Sober, E., & Wilson, D. S. (1999). *Unto others: The evolution and psychology of unselfish behavior.* Harvard University Press.

Solomon, P. (2004). Peer support/peer provided services underlying processes, benefits, and critical ingredients. *Psychiatric Rehabilitation Journal, 27*(4), 392–401. https://doi.org/10.2975/27.2004.392.401

Solomon, P., & Draine, J. (1996). Perspectives concerning consumers as case managers. *Community Mental Health Journal, 32*(1), 41–46. https://doi.org/10.1007/BF02249366

Soto, A., Smith, T. B., Griner, D., Rodriguez, M. D., & Bernal, G. (2019). Cultural adaptations and multicultural competence. In J. C. Norcross & B. E. Wampold (Eds.), *Psychotherapy relationships that work: Volume 2: Evidence-based therapist responsiveness* (3rd ed., Vol. 2, pp. 86–112). Oxford University Press.

Squire, R. W. (1990). A model of empathic understanding and adherence to treatment regimes in practitioner-patient relationships. *Social Science & Medicine, 30*(3), 325–339. https://doi.org/10.1016/0277-9536(90)90188-x

Steadman, H. J. (1992). Boundary spanners: A key component for the effective interactions of the justice and mental health systems. *Law and Human Behavior, 16*(1), 75–87. https://doi.org/10.1007/BF02351050

Stickel, A., Gröpper, S., Pallauf, A., & Goerling, U. (2015). Patients' knowledge and attitudes towards cancer peer support programs. *Oncology, 89*(4), 242–244. https://doi.org/10.1159/000430918

Strohm-Kitchener, K., & Anderson, S. K. (2011). *Foundations of ethical practice, research, and teaching in psychology and counseling* (2nd ed.). Routledge.

Strudwick, G., Zhang, T., Inglis, F., Sockalingam, S., Munnery, M., Lo, B., Takhar, S. S., Charow, R., & Wiljer, D. (2019). Delivery of compassionate mental health care in a digital technology-driven age: Protocol for a scoping review. *BMJ, 9*(7), e027989. http://dx.doi.org/10.1136/bmjopen-2018-027989

Stuart, G. W. (2009). Therapeutic nurse-client relationship. In G. W. Stuart (Ed.), *Principles and practice of psychiatric nursing* (9th ed., pp. 31–38). Mosby.

Stuart, H. (2008). Fighting the stigma caused by mental disorders: Past perspectives, present activities, and future directions. *World Psychiatry, 7*(3), 185–188.

Sucala, M., Schnur, J. B., Brackman, E. H., Constantino, M. J., & Montgomery, G. H. (2013). Clinicians' attitudes toward therapeutic alliance in e-therapy. *Journal of General Psychology, 140*(4), 282–293. https://dx.doi.org/10.1080%2F00221309.2013.830590

Sullivan, H. S. (1952). *The interpersonal theory of psychiatry.* W. W. Norton & Co.

Sunderland, K., Mishkin, W., & Peer Leadership Group, Mental Health Commission of Canada. (2013). *Guidelines for the practice and training of peer support.* Mental Health Commission of Canada. https ://www.mentalhealthcommission.ca/English/document/18291/peer-support-guidelines

Sussman, S. (1998). The first asylums in Canada: A response to neglectful community care and current trends. *Canadian Journal of Psychiatry, 43*(3), 260–264. https://doi.org/10.1177/070674379804300304

Sweeney, A., Fahmy, S., Nolan, F., Morant, N., Fox, Z., Lloyd-Evans, B., Osborn, D., Burgess, E., Gilburt, H., McCabe, R., Slade, M., & Johnson, S. (2014). The relationship between therapeutic alliance and service user satisfaction in mental health inpatient wards and crisis house alternatives: A cross-sectional study. *PloS One, 9*(7), e100153. https://doi.org/10.1371/journal.pone.0100153

Taylor, D., & Bury, M. (2007). Chronic illness, expert patients and care transition. *Sociology of Health & Illness, 29*(1), 27–45.

Tendhar, T. (2019). *Compassion and well-being: The effects of an online film and mediated compassion education on undergraduate students.* Doctoral dissertation. University of Rhode Island Digital Commons. (AAI13877559).

Teplin, L. A., McClelland, G. M., Abram, K. M., & Weiner, D. A. (2006). Crime victimization in adults with severe mental illness: Comparison with the national crime victimization survey. *Archives of General Psychiatry, 62*(8), 911–921. https://dx.doi.org/10.1001%2Farchpsyc.62.8.911

Theodoridou, A., Schlatter, F., Ajdacic, V., Rössler, W., & Jäger, M. (2012). Therapeutic relationship in the context of perceived coercion in a psychiatric population. *Psychiatry Research, 200*(2/3), 939–944. https://doi.org/10.1016/j.psychres.2012.04.012

Thielmann, I., & Hilbig, B. E. (2015). Trust: An integrative review from a person-situation perspective. *Review of General Psychology, 19*(3), 249–277. https://doi.org/10.1037/gpr0000046

Thomas, N., Farhall, J., Foley, F., Rossell, S. L., Castle, D., Ladd, E., Meyer, D., Mihalopolous, C., Leitan, N., Nunan, C., Frankish, R., Smark, T., Farnan, S., McLeod, B., Sterling, L., Murray, G., Fossey, E., Brophy, L., & Kyrios, M. (2016). Randomised controlled trial of a digitally assisted low intensity intervention to promote personal recovery in persisting psychosis: SMART-therapy study protocol. *BMC Psychiatry, 16*(1), 1–12. https://dx.doi.org/10.1186%2Fs12888-016-1024-1

Torous, J., & Hsin, H. (2018). Empowering the digital therapeutic relationship: Virtual clinics for digital health interventions. *NPJ Digital Medicine, 1*(16), 1–3. https://doi.org/10.1038/s41746-018-0028-2

Torous, J., & Roberts, L. W. (2017). The ethical use of mobile health technology in clinical psychiatry. *Journal of Nervous and Mental Disease, 205*(1), 4–8. https://doi.org/10.1097/NMD.0000000000000596

Truax, C. (1961). *A scale for the measurement of accurate empathy.* Wisconsin Psychiatric Institute Paper 20, Madison, WI.

Truax, C. (1970). Effects of client-centred psychotherapy with schizophrenic patients: Nine years pretherapy and nine years posttherapy hospitalization. *Journal of Consulting and Clinical Psychology, 35*(3), 417–422. https://doi.org/10.1037/h0030282

Truax, C. B., & Carkhuff, R. R. (1967). *Towards effective counselling and psychotherapy: Training and practice.* AldineTransaction.

Truax, C., & Mitchell, K. (1971). Research on certain therapist interpersonal skills in relation to process and outcome. In A. Bergin & S. Garfield (Eds.), *Handbook of psychotherapy: An empirical evaluation.* John Wiley.

Tudor, G. E. (1952). A sociopsychiatric nursing approach to intervention in a problem of mutual withdrawal on a mental hospital ward. *Perspectives in Psychiatric Care, 8*(1), 11–35. https://doi.org/10.1111/j.1744-6163.1970.tb01287.x

Tudor, G. E. (1970). A sociopsychiatric nursing approach to intervention in a problem of mutual withdrawal on a mental hospital ward. *Perspectives in Psychiatric Care, 8*(1), 11–35. https://doi.org/10.1111/j.1744-6163.1970.tb01287.x. Reprinted from (1952). *Psychiatry: Journal for the Study of Interpersonal Processes, 15*(2), 193–217. https://doi.org/10.1080/00332747.1952.11022873

Valdesolo, P., & DeSteno, D. (2011). Synchrony and the social tuning of compassion. *Emotion, 11*(2), 262–266. https://doi.org/10.1037/a0021302

Van Kleef, G., van den Berg, H., & Heerdink, M. W. (2015). The persuasive power of emotions: Effects of emotional expressions on attitude formation and change. *Journal of Applied Psychology, 100*(4), 1124–1142. https://psycnet.apa.org/doi/10.1037/apl0000003

Vigo, D., Thornicroft, G., & Atun, R. (2016). Estimating the true global burden of mental illness. *The Lancet Psychiatry, 3*(2), 171–178. https://doi.org/10.1016/S2215-0366(15)00505-2

Vigod, S. N., Kurdyak, P. A., Dennis, C.-L., Leszcz, T., Taylor, V. H., Blumberger, D. M., & Seitz, D. P. (2013). Transitional interventions to reduce early psychiatric readmissions in adults: Systematic review. *British Journal of Psychiatry, 202*(3), 187–194.

Vingilis, E., & Pederson, L. (2001). Using the right tools to answer the right questions: The importance of evaluative research techniques of health services evaluation in the 21st century. *Canadian Journal of Program Evaluation, 16*, 1–26.

Wade, S. L., Raj, S. P., Moscato, E. L., & Narad, M. E. (2019). Clinician perspectives delivering telehealth interventions to children/families impacted by pediatric traumatic brain injury. *Rehabilitation Psychology, 64*(3), 298–306. https://doi.org/10.1037/rep0000268

Wagner, P., Hendrich, J., Moseley, G., & Hudson, V. (2007). Defining medical professionalism: A qualitative study. *Medical Education, 41*(3), 288–294. https://doi.org/10.1111/j.1365-2929.2006.02695.x

Walter, F., Carr, M. J., Mok, P. L., Antonsen, S., Pedersen, C. B., Appleby, L., Fazel, S., Shaw, J., & Webb, R. T. (2019). Multiple adverse outcomes following first discharge from inpatient psychiatric care: A national cohort study. *The Lancet Psychiatry, 6*(7), 582–589. http://dx.doi.org/10.1016/S2215-0366(19)30180-4

Watson, J. (2014). The role of empathy in psychotherapy: Theory, research and practice. In D. Cain, K. Keenan, & S. Rubin (Eds.), *Humanistic psychotherapies: Handbook of research and practice* (pp. 115–145). American Psychological Association.

Weng, H. Y., Fox, A. S., Shackman, A. J., Stodola, D. E., Caldwell, J. Z., Olson, M. C., Rogers, G. M., & Davidson, R. J. (2013). Compassion training alters altruism and neural responses to suffering. *Psychological science, 24*(7), 1171–1180. https://doi.org/10.1177/0956797612469537

Williams, A. (1992). Where has all the empathy gone? *Professional Nurse, 8*(2), 134.

Williams, A., Fossey, E., Farhall, J., Foley, F., & Thomas, N. (2018). Going online together: The potential for mental health workers to integrate recovery oriented e-Mental health resources into their practice. *Psychiatry, 81*(2), 116–129. https://doi.org/10.1080/00332747.2018.1492852

Williams, C. A. (1990). Biopsychosocial elements of empathy: A multidimensional model. *Issues in Mental Health Nursing, 11*(2), 155–174. https://doi.org/10.3109/01612849009014551

Williams, C. L. (1979). Empathic communication and its effect on client outcome. *Issues in Mental Health Nursing, 2*(1), 15–26. https://doi.org/10.3109/01612847909058196

World Health Organization. (2020). *eHealth at WHO.* https://www.who.int/ehealth/about/en/

Wright, K., & McKeown, M. (Eds.). (2018). *Essentials of mental health nursing.* SAGE Publications Ltd.

Yu, J., & Kirk, M. (2009). Evaluation of empathy measurement tools in nursing: Systematic review. *Journal of Advanced Nursing, 65*(9), 1790–1806. https://doi.org/10.1111/j.1365-2648.2009.05071.x

Index

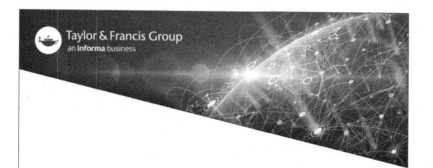

ted in the United States
Bookmasters